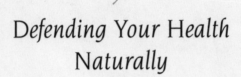

Defending Your Health
Naturally

Defending Your Health Naturally

FIVE LINES OF DEFENSE TO IMPROVE HEALTH AND INCREASE STAMINA

*

Louis Vanrenen

JEREMY P. TARCHER/PENGUIN
a member of Penguin Group (USA) Inc.

JEREMY P. TARCHER/PENGUIN

Published by the Penguin Group

Penguin Group (USA) Inc., 375 Hudson Street, New York,
New York 10014, USA • Penguin Group (Canada), 90 Eglinton Avenue East, Suite 700,
Toronto, Ontario M4P 2Y3, Canada, (a division of Pearson Penguin Canada Inc.) • Penguin
Books Ltd, 80 Strand, London WC2R 0RL, England • Penguin Ireland, 25 St Stephen's Green,
Dublin 2, Ireland (a division of Penguin Books Ltd) • Penguin Group (Australia), 250 Camber-
well Road, Camberwell, Victoria 3124, Australia (a division of Pearson Australia Group Pty Ltd)
• Penguin Books India Pvt Ltd, 11 Community Centre, Panchsheel Park, New Delhi–110 017,
India • Penguin Group (NZ), Cnr Airborne and Rosedale Roads, Albany, Auckland 1310,
New Zealand (a division of Pearson New Zealand Ltd) • Penguin Books (South Africa) (Pty)
Ltd, 24 Sturdee Avenue, Rosebank, Johannesburg 2196, South Africa

Penguin Books Ltd., Registered Offices: 80 Strand, London WC2R 0RL, England

An application has been submitted to register this book with the Library of Congress.
ISBN 1-58542-417-X

Printed in the United States of America
1   3   5   7   9   10   8   6   4   2

BOOK DESIGN BY TANYA MAIBORODA

Neither the publisher nor the author is engaged in rendering professional advice or services to the
individual reader. The ideas, procedures, and suggestions contained in this book are not intended
as a substitute for consulting with your physician. All matters regarding your health require medical supervision. Neither the author nor the publisher shall be liable or responsible for any loss or
damage allegedly arising from any information or suggestion in this book.

While the author has made every effort to provide accurate telephone numbers and Inter-
net addresses at the time of publication, neither the publisher nor the author assumes any
responsibility for errors, or for changes that occur after publication. Further, the publisher does
not have any control over and does not assume any responsibility for author or third-party web-
sites or their content.

Most Tarcher/Penguin books are available at special quantity discounts for bulk purchase
for sales promotions, premiums, fund-raising, and educational needs. Special books or book
excerpts also can be created to fit specific needs. For details, write Penguin Group (USA) Inc. Special Markets, 375 Hudson Street, New York, NY 10014.

To Gabriel and Ariana Vanrenen,
my son and daughter

Contents

Appendixes

Defending Your Health Naturally

Introduction

THE IDEA FOR THIS BOOK, AND ITS CORE INFORMATION—
the five lines of defense—derive from years of experience
with Oriental and nutritional medicine. Recently, a wealth of
information about diet and nutrition has permeated American
consciousness. Research into plant constituents and healthful
foods has resulted in a quiet revolution. The old adage "Food
is your best medicine" is now proving its worth. We now
know that certain foods can help prevent disease, even such
formidable diseases as cancer.

Oriental medicine is an ancient tradition with a continu-
ous history of more than two thousand years. This holistic

practice combines an array of methods and ideas to promote health and treat disease: acupuncture, bodywork, herbal medicine, dietetics, and a dazzling array of healthful exercises. The system is ably designed to support the whole person, prevent disease, and promote health. In Oriental medicine the body is one, energized by a vital energy, and all physical symptoms are intimately related to our vitality, which is intimately connected to our emotional/mental life. Preserving and nourishing vitality is the core of Oriental medical practices, whether through the use of medicines, foods, or exercises.

The concept that food is a medicine, a practice that is still breaking into contemporary medicine, is one of the foundations of Oriental medicine. Western culture is still burdened by the assumption that this ancient practice is filled with interesting ideas but little real practical wisdom. Oriental herbalists have successfully been using herbs and food to treat a wide range of diseases for centuries, even bacterial and viral infections. The experience and practicality of this venerable system are undeniable.

One could say that Western medicine is still young when it comes to health promotion and disease prevention. While the incredible achievements of the surgery and drugs of Western medicine cannot be denied, the goal of Eastern and other traditional systems from around the planet has always been preserving the gift of health, supporting the body, and nourishing the spirit. The health of the individual is intimately connected to the vital energy, to his or her immediate society, and to the planet as a whole. In these times of stress and anxiety, there is an imperative to turn to the innate intelligence of nature, which is in our bodies and all around us. This deep respect for the body and methods to support it are at the heart of this book. This approach derives from the web of healing around the planet: modern scientific research, nutritional science, Oriental medicine, European naturopathic traditions, global herbal medicine, and the spiritual traditions of all cultures.

CHAPTER 1

How This Book Can Help You
Defend Your Health

THIS BOOK CAN HELP YOU BECOME MORE ENERGETIC AND healthy. Simple methods that defend health and prevent disease can be incorporated into daily life. Our health is a precious gift, our most important resource. Good health is founded on vitality. For centuries, Asians have called vitality *chi*. Chi is the basis of health. It is the force that gives life and provides abundant energy. Without vitality we are tired, anxious, and prone to illness. We cannot sleep well, and our day is marked by periods of lethargy. We artificially boost our body with too much caffeine, fats, and sugar—all stimulants—and these in

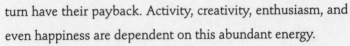

turn have their payback. Activity, creativity, enthusiasm, and even happiness are dependent on this abundant energy.

Imagine that our body is a lightbulb. When the light is on, the whole bulb is infused with energy and light. Light radiates around the bulb. Our physical energy can be compared to a pulsating light that fills our body. There is a natural rhythm of this energy through the day, with slight fluctuations, but essentially it keeps us going until night, when it becomes quiescent. At night the energy is allowed to rejuvenate, getting us ready for another day. For many of us, however, the energy dips down too much, and we feel tired, lethargic, and depressed. For various reasons, often a variety of life stresses, the bulb becomes dimmer. This is not so bad if it rebounds in a few hours or the next day—as it often does—but if this low-grade energy persists day after day it is not good. Our vitality becomes sluggish. We feel irritable and fatigued. Our potential for happiness and friendship diminishes. Our enthusiasm for work and play sags. In time we become more susceptible to colds, viruses, and other health problems.

It is a well-known fact that a tired and lethargic body can compromise the immune system. Our prime defense against disease agents cannot work efficiently. Virus, bacteria, and even cancer can then become more active. Each healthy person's body contains bacteria, viruses, and cancer cells, but these potential terrorists are kept in check by the strong arms of the immune system. Little armies of immune cells surge through the blood and gobble up harmful disease agents. One branch of the immune system even has cells that insert chemicals into foreign cells and kill them. Nasty viruses and other toxins can be eliminated before they spread and overwhelm the immune response. Indeed, this happens every day in the incredible factory of our energy machine, the human body.

Defending our health means supporting the energy and functions of the body. With simple, natural, safe methods, we can promote a vigorous, healthy body. Clear and practical strategies will be presented that allow readers to gain more power over their health. We don't need to rely on medications as much. While we need doctor's visits, we can use the doctor's help in our program to defend our health. Our Western medical system focuses on treating disease, the result of poor vitality and resistance. We even see it in the word: disease. Oriental medicine, the product of many centuries, offers simple methods to promote health and thus *prevent* the onset of disease. While health can never be perfect, we can become stronger and more vigorous by listening to the needs of the marvelous engine, the human body.

During the past decade there has been a quiet revolution in health care, a movement toward more responsible and intelligent self-care. Oriental and ancient holistic methods and ideas have permeated American society. The best of these strategies can be easily incorporated into our lives. While Western medicine, with all its skills and knowledge, has focused on treating disease, Oriental medicine emphasizes health promotion and disease prevention. The best of both worlds is offered in this book. The heart of this book is a practical guide to health promotion. Offered is a range of strategies: therapeutic foods and herbs, specific exercises, and commonsense health tips.

DO YOU FEEL TIRED ALL THE TIME?

There are many unpleasant symptoms that plague people every day: fatigue, headaches, irritability, and fluctuations of energy. Many people suffer too much from sagging energy, which can in time produce moderate depression, malaise, and apathy. Are pills going to help this state? Much of the time, pills will not help. They might even hinder the natural balance of potential health. Certainly if our doctor diagnoses a specific disease and advises a medication, this can be necessary. But much of the time this low-grade health puzzles doctors and they don't have much to offer. In Oriental medicine, this kind of low-grade health can be a precursor to more serious health problems. Many people who have developed obesity, depression, and migraines first experienced a long period of poor energy.

Poor-quality energy and sluggishness can aggravate worry. People become less efficient in life. The quality of their play and work time suffers. In this unpleasant cycle the mind worries about health, which in turn affects the health. When the engine of the body is running poorly, all its functions can suffer. We are more prone to colds and allergies. We can suffer from headaches and poor memory and a loss of focus. We are more susceptible to fluctuations in mood, to anxiety and fussing about insignificant things. When the energy is low, there is not enough vigor for enjoyment and intimacy. Happiness and joy are dependent on abundant energy.

Poor-quality energy can result in the following problems and diseases:

Fatigue
Periods of tiredness and malaise
Poor memory
Moodiness
Low sex drive
Obesity
Depression and anxiety
Diabetes
Heart problems
Susceptibility to colds and flu
Stress-related diseases

Many common problems and diseases are preventable. The average person can be more energetic and healthy. Vigor can result in greater happiness and success. Remember that money is a form of energy. Physical energy and vigor can bring us the money we need to be happy and satisfied. Scientific research tells us that many diseases are preventable. Even certain cancers. Health habits and certain foods can prevent many kinds of cancer and other life-threatening diseases.

THE ENERGY MACHINE

How can we take charge of our health? How can we improve the fundamental fact of health: abundant vitality?

The body is an incredibly complex energy machine. Every cell has the components to convert basic chemicals into energy, which then activates all the organs and glands of the body. This incredible machine is then ready to do its daily work with vigor and consistency. Every body is given a daily allotment of energy. The quality of this energy differs from person to person. Genetics and body type have a role in determining energy levels. Lifestyle and nutrition are equally important. For some people the energy is abundant. Some average five hours of sleep a night and then go through the day like dynamos. They are a minority. Other people have adequate energy, but they must pace themselves. Many people, however, suffer from fluctuations of energy, up and down like a seesaw. Little problems become big, work a chore, and fun and enjoyment distant goals.

Each day, there is a renewal of this energy during sleep. For many, seven or eight hours are sufficient. The food we eat contains energy, which the body absorbs. The air we breathe is important for the energy machine. Another overlooked source of energy is right in front of us: our friends, activities, and entertainment. We all know certain people who are good to be around. Generally, they have abundant energy. Friendships can give us energy. Our jobs can be a significant source of life. Certain activities nourish body and soul: walking the beach, dancing, baseball, playing with children, music, prayer, and meditation. Each day the remarkable energy machine absorbs and expends energy. Defending our health means nourishing the energy machine so that there is not a serious deficit at the end of the week.

Vitality Index

What are your energy levels?

* Do you feel energetic all day?
* Do you wake up alert and vigorous?
* Do you sleep well?
* Do you express enthusiasm each day—about work, play, or hobbies?
* Do you not get annoying minor ailments like colds?

If you answered a big yes to all the above, you are a lucky person. You are blessed with extraordinary vitality. Nourish it! Of course, other factors come into play in creating this excellent energy vitality index: genetics, family, attitudes. But the bottom line in daily life is the levels of physical energy. Just as a car will not run without gas, we do not run without this essential energy. Most of us are not so consistent. We might answer yes to some of the questions. And there will be some who are responding negatively to all the questions. However, it is important to emphasize that the vitality index is not a measure of perfection. Not all of us can feel vigorous and energetic all day long every day of the week. We should not feel guilty because we didn't get a perfect score! But for most of us there is one undeniable fact, good news in fact. We can support and nourish the physical energy of the body, enhance the energy, and promote better health.

A big step toward more consistent energy is our daily food, the quality of the fuel we put into our bodies each day. Sadly, in America today much of this food is devitalizing. We need to consume energizing foods and avoid the cheap sources of fuel so prevalent in this fast-food nation. America is becoming a fat and sedentary nation, plagued by diseases that are often marked by inflammation.

SUPPORTING THE BODY AND MIND

There are many ways to defend your health. There are many ways to increase energy. In later chapters we will discuss essential ways in more detail: super foods and herbs, special exercises, and other health tips. But it is important at this point to emphasize that the path to better health does have a variety of directions. Bicycling or running nourishes some people. Others enjoy games with friends or different kinds of music. Many seek out periods of solitude and prayer. Whatever methods we use to nourish the soul and body, all of us live in a body. This incredible machine with its extraordinary talent for activity is an animal, and that animal thrives on movement: walking, running, stretching, swimming, dancing, and many other kinds. The body is a marvelous animal machine: limbs, joints, blood, and nerves, one dynamic whole. All the parts and the whole thrive on movement: Blood flows better, muscles are invigorated, joints are stretched, and the mind becomes more active. Sluggishness and sedentary life diminish the circulation of blood and energy through the body.

As a baseline, each person should devote at least half an hour each day to the body, a special time set aside for treating this vehicle well. After all, we live in our bodies every day. They need our care and support. Each of us needs to find those activities that our bodies enjoy. Enjoyment of movement is energizing. People with a passion for dance, for instance, are transported away. Their bodies are living well. A mixture of activities is best—walking for half an hour one day, maybe some sport on another. Some people enjoy specific exercises such as those found in the gym or yoga studio. But there is one kind of exercise that all can benefit from: a short amount of stretching. Limbs, joints, and the spine really benefit from just a little stretching every day. This allows the body to be more relaxed and free. Cats know this instinctively. Stretching and flowing physical movement allows the physical energy to be more abundant. Tensions and constrictions can be released. In Oriental medicine, one of the foundations of health is freedom of movement of the natural energy in the limbs and spine, as well as inside the organs, chest, and abdomen. Various tensions can develop in the abdomen or chest. These chronic constrictions result in disease predisposition, such as poor breathing, digestive troubles, even mood changes. In a later section, simple basic stretches will be explained: a simple routine that can be incorporated into daily life with no fuss. We call this an essential part of the body tune-up.

Our mind and emotions also need to be fed and nourished. Of course, they affect the health of the energy of the physical body. Once again, activities of the mind and heart are dependent on each person. One has to listen to one's needs, what calls you in life. Some people like to study sports or history, others like games or song. Many find that setting aside a part of each day for prayer, contemplation, or meditation is nourishing. Sometimes it is important to spend a short time of the day doing nothing. Relaxation is fundamental, but too much downtime can be spent watching TV or playing on the computer. A little of this time could be set aside for a more substantial body or soul exercise.

SUMMING UP

The incredible machine of the body can be supported and nourished so that its physical energy is stronger and more resilient. Defending our health means active involvement in health promotion: This is not a great chore. It does not take up so much time. This book introduces simple methods that can promote health and prevent disease. We all can learn specific tools and strategies for addressing specific problems like colds, backache, or arthritis—the theme of chapter 4.

However, before introducing the core of this book, there is one short chapter on factors that deplete energy and cause disease. In order to defend our health, there are certain facts that we need to know. What is the root of pain? Why is it that some people never get colds? What is it that causes so many inflammatory diseases that plague Americans: arthritis, tendinitis, carpal tunnel syndrome, migraines, and back pain? How can we avoid disease? Many disease states begin from several changes in the overall operation of the body, and when we recognize these we can take better charge of our health.

CHAPTER 2

Reducing Stress:
A Pathway to Better Health

PAIN AND MANY HEALTH PROBLEMS RESULT FROM SEVERAL interrelated factors that we can control. As was said in the first chapter, vitality is the root of health. What are the factors that deplete energy and lead to dis-ease? Many experts recognize that a common cause of poor health and many diseases is stress or, we might say, excess stress.

Stress is a normal part of life—in fact, a necessary part. We cannot do without some stress in life. Some stresses are challenging and invigorating. We might have a problem in our daily work, but when we have solved it we feel satisfied and proud. However, in busy modern life we are inundated with a wide variety of stresses that are not rewarding and energizing. All the chemicals in our environment and foods are stresses to the body. In the past fifty years, thousands of new and sometimes toxic chemicals have been introduced into our food, air, and water. Too much electromagnetic pollution is another stress to the vitality. Cell phones, computer screens, and television sets surround us. Other common forms of stress include overwork, emotional trauma, and lack of adequate sleep. Prolonged arguments and conflicts are a profound form of potentially debilitating stress. Thinking too much can be de-energizing. We have all had the experience of mulling things over too much and worrying about the past or future. Living in the present is not an easy task.

Too much sitting is another form of stress. The body becomes lazy and lethargic. Some people sit all day at work, sit in their cars on the way home, and then plunk themselves in front of the TV for the evening, before lying down for eight hours! It is therapeutic to inject some body tune-up time into that busy but sedentary schedule.

Henry James, the esteemed American philosopher, once said that will is volitional. We can make choices. We can pay close and compassionate attention to our mind and body states. We can work to live more in the present. This light of attention is one of the great benefits of a life well lived.

Another fundamental source of stress is the curious diet

that many Americans have adopted: fried foods, sugar, nutritionally depleted processed food, and too much meat. Once in a while during the week we can enjoy French fries, a hamburger or a pizza, or some potato chips, but we have to realize that fast food is de-energizing. It overloads the body, taxes the liver, and inhibits the proper utilization of good nutrients. It saps the energy machine. It should not be our regular diet.

Our instinct for real, whole, and vitalized food has suffered in the past decades. Just as the body has a need for healthy movement, it has a need for vitalizing, nourishing foods. The body flourishes on fresh nutrients from vegetables, fruits, and whole grains—far more nourishing than white flour—and it needs small amounts of good-quality protein—a sensible balance of fish, eggs, cheese, and lean meat. Because the basic diet of so many Americans is de-energizing, they turn to cheap sources of quick energy: sugar, caffeine, fats, and lots of greasy meat. This inevitably creates a sluggish body and person. In the next chapter we will discuss the basis of a healthy diet that energizes and prolongs life. This diet is simple and reasonable, not a burden, and can be an investment into longevity and vigor. We can still enjoy the many good things of life like coffee, wine, pizza, bagels, and, yes, cheesecake. But these luxury foods exist as a special treat against the background of daily nourishing foods, the whole-foods diet.

Common Sources of Stress That Can in Time Compromise Energy and Health

❋ Overwork: Too many long hours, not enough relaxation time.

❋ Not enough sleep or restless sleep night after night.

❋ Mental/emotional distress: Everyone can have emotional distress, but when it goes on day after day, it begins to create a big leak in the energy machine.

❋ A sloppy junk-food diet, day after day, with no real foods. (The long-term adverse effects of this diet will be examined in a later chapter.)

❋ Too many chemicals: Synthetic chemicals are in our foods, air, water, carpets, and medicines. Chemicals overload the liver and toxify the body. Some specific foods and herbs will be presented that can help the body eliminate this toxic overload.

❋ Sedentary: Not enough simple and even short-term exercise.

❋ Electromagnetic pollution: Ever felt exhausted after several hours in front of the computer or television screen?

❋ Emotional trauma, mental anguish: We cannot avoid it if our grandmother dies or we lose our job because of downsizing. However, we can use methods presented in this book to support the body and soul in these trying times.

✳ Negative attitudes: In various ways this key topic is the subject of many books. One simple term for bad attitude is "'life sucks' syndrome." It has many variations and themes—guilt, jealousy, anger, apathy—but the bottom line is that it drains the life energy of the body. For each person, one of life's purposes is to struggle against our particular brand of "life sucks" attitude.

Bottom Line

Excess and prolonged stresses deplete the energy and overtax the body. The multiple and prolonged stresses of modern life are like leaks in the marvelous energy machine. There are simple solutions to mitigate the multiple effects of life stresses—read on. Our ability to defend our health improves when we come to a better understanding of how excess stress harms the body. What exactly does it do, and more important, what can we do to help the body?

STRESS, THE SOURCE OF MANY DISEASES

Research and observation clearly indicate that stress can deplete the body's energy, overtax the organs and glands, and overwork the nervous system. Excess and prolonged stress causes a cascade of chemical reactions in the body. One example is the so-called fight-or-flight response, which results in a release of powerful hormones from the adrenal glands. Stress hits, and bang, the chemical response inundates the body, enabling it to battle the real or imaginary threat. One stress hormone, cortisol, raises blood sugar for increased energy. Once the perceived threat has passed, the chemicals linger in the body. Excess cortisol leads to excess blood sugar, which then has to be stored as fat. Studies have found that women with high levels of body fat accumulating at their waist also have high levels of cortisol in their system due to elevated levels of stress. Up-and-down swings of blood sugar due to cortisol also promote food cravings and a sugary diet, which can then turn simple weight problems into diabetes— a classic disease involving inflammation, stress, and diet.

One other insidious result from stress and poor diet is a gradual, barely perceptible generalized inflammatory response, which in turn makes us susceptible to arthritis, cancer, Alzheimer's disease, or coronary heart disease. In turn, this can lead to an overactive immune response. Confused by the internal inflammation, the immune system attacks parts of the body. If this happens in the blood vessels, damage to the arteries can ensue, a potential cause of coronary heart disease.

It is important to emphasize that much short-term pain is

caused by localized inflammation, an actual healing response to injury. When we fall and twist our ankle, the tissue around the joint swells up, and that hurts. This is localized inflammation. The generalized internal inflammation we are now speaking of is potentially harmful and can lead to chronic disease.

While the inflammatory factor is not yet fully recognized by conventional medicine, many nutritionist and holistic researchers are recognizing the broad role that stress, faulty diet, and inflammation play in many diseases. Oriental medicine, however, has long understood this triad of disease genesis. In Oriental medicine, inflammation is called overheating and has three pathways in the body: toxification, pain, and disease; overstimulation of the nervous system, which leads to nervousness, anxiety, hyperactivity, and abnormal sweating; irritability and tension, which leads to muscular constriction and headaches.

DISEASES RELATED TO HIGH STRESS AND SUBSEQUENT INFLAMMATION

* High blood pressure (Primary hypertension can often be moderated by a good diet and stress reduction.)
* Diabetes
* Arthritis
* Autoimmune diseases

* Ulcers
* Some kinds of cancer
* Pain and inflammation
* Obesity
* Colitis

Unfortunately, the effects of excess stress are numerous. One major result is toxic overload of the body. The body becomes inundated with too many chemicals and free radicals, overtaxing the liver, the main organ that cleans the blood of toxins and chemicals. The liver becomes less efficient, leading to a prolonged low-grade dysfunction, which does not necessarily reflect in blood tests. The result is that the body becomes more susceptible to disease factors like virus and bacteria.

Toxic overload is not a condition that can be easily diagnosed. It is not a disease, but it can most definitely lead to disease. How do you know you have it? Many symptoms can indicate some degree of toxic overload: headaches, fatigue, irritability, swollen glands, poor digestion, constipation, diarrhea, swollen or stiff joints, and just plain feeling lousy much of the time.

The good news is that we can reduce toxic overload and inflammation. We can rid the body of conditions that lead to disease. We can rid the body of pain.

FREE RADICALS, ANTIOXIDANTS, AND THE LIVER

These topics may sound intimidating, even boring, but in exploring them we can learn fascinating information about how disease takes hold in the body. We can also learn how to help the body, to defend our health.

FREE RADICALS

During cellular work, the body produces wastes, including free radicals that enter the bloodstream somewhat like terrorists. Free radicals, which also come from the environment, are one of the underlying causes of aging and the inception of many chronic degenerative diseases—cancer, heart failure, and arthritis. Dr. Roy L. Walford, the author of *Maximum Lifespan,* explains the role of free radicals in the body.

> Another and equally destructive class of damaging agents produced during metabolism but present in the environment as well are the free radicals. . . . Great white sharks in the biochemical sea, these short-lived but voracious agents oxidize and damage tissue.[1]

Dr. Walford explains that if our body did not neutralize free radicals, we would become solid, as we do in rigor mortis

[1]Dr. Roy L. Walford, *Maximum Lifespan* (New York: W. W. Norton, 1985).

when we die. In fact, we would plasticize. Free radical technology forms the basis of the modern plastics industry. Our environment and modern lifestyle now generate more free radicals than in the past.

When the body becomes overly toxic, it can no longer adequately neutralize and eliminate poisons, cellular debris, free radicals, and other constituents that compromise vital functions. This overload of toxins compromises both the liver and immune system, leading to sluggish functions, malaise, and low-key inflammations, which in turn lead to disease and premature aging. In his book *Food as Medicine,* Dr. Dharma Singh Khalsa says, "The negative signals received by DNA from free radicals may also cause the production of other chemicals such as prostaglandins, which create the inflammation that leads to arthritis and many other illnesses, including Alzheimer's.[2] Dr. Khalsa lists diseases that are related to chronic inflammation and toxification. These include cancer, heart attack, arthritis, fibromyalgia, and allergies. Unfortunately, Dr. Khalsa is among a tiny minority in the medical profession: He is well aware of the link connecting foods, stress reduction, and vigorous health. His training included nutrition

[2]Dharma Singh Khalsa, *Food as Medicine: How to Use Diet, Vitamins, Juices, and Herbs for a Healthier, Happier, and Longer Life* (New York: Atria Books, 2003), p. 17.

Inflammation Syndrome and Modern Medicine

Some readers are probably asking, "Is all this talk about inflammation and disease a bunch of nonsense?" Nutritional research is the forefront of these ideas and is beginning to infiltrate established medicine. From the March 8, 2003, *Time* magazine article about diabetes: "Over the past five years, researchers have shown that inflammation is at least as important as high cholesterol in causing heart disease. . . . Could the same be true for diabetes?"

and ecology of the body, not subjects emphasized in medical school. Dr. Khalsa goes on to explain another intriguing fact: Low-grade inflammatory conditions make us more susceptible to the flu virus, harmful bacteria, and other virulent disease agents. As he explains, this susceptibility can be decreased with good foods, herbal medicines, and antioxidants.

Why do some people never get the flu even if they work in an office full of sick people? Symptoms of the flu are signs of inflammation and immune reaction. With some people, the immune system and cleansing functions of the body work together to produce a state of vigor and adaptation.

In diseases like arthritis, inflammation plays a major destructive role, involving a cascade of chemical effects that is partly instigated by an enzyme, COX-2. Recent publicity about the negative effects of many major arthritic drugs only highlights our need to return to simple natural methods of inflammation reduction: healthful foods, herbal medicines, and exercise.

Many herbs, like turmeric and ginger, can safely moderate inflammation, pain, and disease. These herbs are notable also because they do not have the side effects of pharmaceutical anti-inflammatory drugs. In fact, some researchers believe that some medical drugs—particularly those used for pain reduction—can in the long run aggravate inflammation. Many common foods also can inhibit inflammation. Equally important is to avoid proinflammatory foods, a subject discussed in the next chapter. How can we neutralize free radicals, those nasty terrorists that can at times run rampant in our blood and cells? One answer is simple: consuming the antioxidants found in many vegetables, seeds, herbs, and grains.

ANTIOXIDANTS

Antioxidants, constituents of numerous foods and herbs, help to neutralize excess free radicals. They also can decrease inflammation, support the immune system, and help the body defend itself from disease. Plants, like humans, are susceptible to bacteria, viruses, and cancer. Free radicals, the rogue molecules, can also adversely affect plants. However, plants contain phytochemicals, antioxidants that can neutralize these free radicals. What is even more interesting is that these antioxidants can also inhibit disease agents like bacteria and cancer cells. Dr. Thomas Slaga, a pioneer in the research of beneficial plant constituents, and other researchers have determined that constituents in plants assist the liver in detoxification and neutralize harmful free radicals, as well as enhance the functioning of the immune system.

This trio of therapeutic functions is truly remarkable and can have profound effects on our health. One could cite many examples. The phytochemical D-glucarate (found in broccoli, cabbage, Brussels sprouts, apples, apricots, and other fruits) detoxifies chemicals that can lead to certain kinds of cancer. Green tea contains constituents that we now know can inhibit cancer cells, harmful bacteria, and viruses.[3] Many constituents of all plants have the potential to neutralize free radicals and reduce toxic inflammations. Quercetin, now available in supplement form, is a very common phytochemical found in countless plants. Quercetin is one of nature's safest anti-inflammatory substances, and many physicians trained in nutrition use it, often with vitamin C, to treat injuries and

[3]Thomas Slaga, *The Detox Revolution* (New York: McGraw-Hill, 2003), p. 11.

A Short List of Major Phytochemica

Many herbs are particularly rich in phytochemicals, but as we can see they are also found in fruits and vegetables. Herbal medicines differ from healthful foods in that they contain more specific and concentrated healing components. Pharmaceutical drugs do not contain any nutrients, phytochemicals, or vitamins because they are isolated and purified chemicals.

Many vegetables and herbs contain antioxidants that protect the body from cancer, harmful bacteria, and pernicious virus. Common antioxidants include carotenoids, flavonoids, indoles, saponins, and terpenes. While these names might be strange to most people, their healing potential is diverse, practical, and potent. Scientists have found, for example, that the indoles in kale and cabbage can actually block cancer-causing substances from activating in the body. Other antioxidants inhibit the activity of harmful disease agents, heal damaged tissue, and improve blood circulation.

promote general health. Phytochemicals are also healthy for the heart, liver, and blood vessels.

Bottom Line

Enjoy a wide variety of fruits and vegetables in a range of colors since these indicate different antioxidants. There are sixty kinds of fruits on the market. Most Americans eat six. Be adventurous. Try all the colors: orange, red, yellow, green, purple. An important tip: The darker the green vegetable, the more nourishing it is. Overlooked vegetables like kale, Brussels sprouts, collard greens, and watercress are extraordinarily abundant in a range of therapeutic constituents.

Many people now recognize that antioxidants are good for health, and they rush out to purchase an expensive bottle of vitamins. It is not enough to add antioxidant vitamins to our diet. One has to eliminate those chemicals that cause the damage in the first place. Common sense cries out that adding good fuel to a dirty, sluggish engine is not rational. One important step in the healing process is to be kind to the poor overworked liver, one of the most stressed organs in the modern world.

Some readers might be skeptical about these conclusions. But the facts are there, and for the most part they are both enlightening and astounding. Simple plants, taken for granted, contain therapeutic chemicals that disarm free radicals, cancer, bacteria, and viruses. With safe plant medicines we now have the potential to inhibit noxious bacteria and other disease agents. We now have the knowledge to assist the healing powers of the body with simple, safe methods. The use of chemical drugs can be decreased. The ecology of the body, not to mention our well-being, will be greatly assisted by this knowledge.

THE LIVER AND DETOXIFICATION

The most important organ for "cleaning" the blood is the liver, which is aided by the intestines, kidneys, and lymph and immune systems. The liver is an immensely important organ with numerous vital functions. For example, it stores vitamins and releases them into the body when needed. At night, while we rest, the liver releases hormones that travel through the body, restoring and reviving cells. The liver is also a highly intelligent organ, a cleaning house for environmental toxins, chemical poisons, and by-products of cellular work. Poor and inefficient liver functioning, while not a disease, can compromise general health and vitality and lay the groundwork for many diseases. Poor liver function may be accompanied by such symptoms as mood changes, tiredness, irritability, and headaches.

One of the recent breakthroughs in the scientific understanding of the body has been the role of the liver in detoxification of chemicals and toxins. A key two-step process has been identified whereby potent chemicals can be effectively neutralized and eliminated. Though this process can occur in cells throughout the body, the center of action is the remarkable liver. When a harmful chemical enters the body, it must go through the liver. The liver recognizes and targets these noxious substances, which can be seemingly benign substances such as aspirin. In a two-step process, liver enzymes disarm the chemicals and convert them into harmless substances. This complex process goes on all the time with the many harmful chemicals in our foods, drugs, and air, and even by-products of work in the body. It is absolutely vital for general health that the liver work efficiently. In many people, this system of detoxification becomes sluggish and inefficient, leading to headaches, fatigue, malaise, bad temper, and even predisposition to diseases like cancer. It is important to emphasize that elevated levels of specific wastes in the blood can lead to diseases like cancer. Scientific researchers like Dr. Slaga emphasize that the efficient two-phase detoxification strategy of the liver is central to good health. Furthermore, these researchers emphasize that phytochemicals in foods and herbs help the liver in its essential role of detoxification. This groundbreaking research is very recent, within the last decade, and introduces a whole new element into modern medicine: prevention and treatment of disease with foods and medicinal plants.

Incredibly enough, there is increasing evidence that some constituents in foods and herbal medicines can heal damaged

DNA. When DNA is damaged by viruses, chemicals, and other insults, the potential for cancer increases dramatically. Countless constituents of all plants have the potential to neutralize free radicals and reduce toxic inflammations. Already mentioned is quercetin, which is found in many plants and herbs. Quercetin, along with other phytochemicals, is also healthy for the heart, liver, and blood vessels. Even more interesting is the potential of some herbal medicines to assist the body to eliminate toxins and poisons. Research is making it increasingly evident that herbs like turmeric, milk thistle, and schisandra have multiple healing functions in the body. Researchers have determined that this remarkable trio of herbs assists the efficient detoxifying processes of the liver. Furthermore, it is evident that these herbs can even heal liver cells that have been damaged by exposure to drugs and environmental chemicals. For those interested in more details, consult *The Detox Revolution* by Dr. Thomas Slaga.

SUMMING UP

We see that the triad of excess stress, toxification, and inflammation are fundamental sources of discomfort and pain. They result in diminished vitality, lethargy, and susceptibility to disease. Low-grade energy becomes the daily norm, and disease predisposition is activated. The body is then susceptible to internal disharmonies, manifesting in headaches, swelling, aches, flu, and digestive troubles, and it cannot defend itself against harmful bacteria, nasty viruses, and cancer.

The good news is that we can address these problems with simple, practical strategies that can be easily incorporated into daily life. We can take charge of our health. We don't have to be at the mercy of disease agents. We don't have to rely on pharmaceutical drugs as much. It is sad to say, but the abuse of chemical drugs, so common nowadays, adds to the toxification of the body. Even relatively benign drugs like Tylenol are hard on the liver and must be broken down and eliminated. While medical checkups and tests are always important, we can trust the healing wisdom of our own bodies. We can help the body to do what it has always done quite well: heal itself.

The following chapter will present the five lines of defense, a unique system to prevent disease and promote health.

CHAPTER 3

The Five Lines of Defense

THIS CHAPTER IS THE HEART OF THIS BOOK. HOW CAN WE defend our health? The vital energy of good health is protected by five lines of defense, a synthesis of Eastern and Western concepts of health promotion. These five lines of defense can be summarized as:

1. Promoting health and energy. Our daily energy depends on our basic fuel, our daily diet.

2. Stress reduction. Reducing stress takes a load off the body—the nervous and hormonal systems—and provides more energy for living.

3. Detoxification, or cleansing and elimination. Toxins and harmful chemicals can come from both outside of the body— most notably synthetic chemicals—and inside. Just as a car produces exhaust from the burning of gas, the millions of cells in our bodies produce waste from chemical work. Excess stresses in life can add to the chemical overload of the body. Furthermore, wastes and unusable matter from our food must be expelled in the stools or urine.

4. Decreasing inflammation. As stated in the last chapter, generalized inflammation is a common background in many diseases.

5. The immune system. Our primary defense against disease agents is like a sword and shield. When it is functioning well and efficiently, we are less likely to contract viral diseases, bacterial infections, and cancer.

LINE OF DEFENSE 1:
PROMOTING HEALTH AND ENERGY

As was said in the first chapter, health is dependent on good energy. To put it another way, vitality is the foundation of health. While we cannot quantify vitality, either with a machine or test tube, common sense informs us that we have an energy that fuels us. Biochemists call this basic energy ATP. ATP is made in the furnace of each of the millions of cells in our bodies—the mitochondria. Physicians practicing Oriental

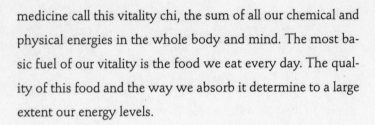

medicine call this vitality chi, the sum of all our chemical and physical energies in the whole body and mind. The most basic fuel of our vitality is the food we eat every day. The quality of this food and the way we absorb it determine to a large extent our energy levels.

Daily Food and Nutrition

Our basic energy for daily living and good health comes from the food we consume each day. Our body is not a simple combustion engine. The machine of our body is extraordinarily complex, but it can work very well for many years. We can increase our daily energy, enthusiasm, and stamina with good, nourishing foods.

We often use the term "diet" to mean a special regime to lose weight. In this book, diet connotes our daily fare. The guidelines that follow are not specifically for losing weight, though they will help. They are a general strategy for everyone— what to eat, what to avoid, how to stay healthy and vigorous with the right fuel. Later in the book there is a separate section on weight loss.

Despite the many diets, fads, and books, there is no mystery anymore about what constitutes a healthy diet for all Americans. Many authorities and experts recognize this diet plan now, after years of confused advice. However, it is important to emphasize that there is no perfect daily food program for everyone. The guidelines offered are a good foundation. People have slightly different nutritional profiles. For example, those who are very active require more protein in the form of meat, eggs, and fish. Those who have specific medical problems might require a specific nutritional plan. Guidelines offered are based on centuries of experiences and modern research, but we should be adaptable and sometimes seek out professional advice.

The advice recommended in this book is based on Oriental medicine and many modern nutrition experts. For a positive model we can also turn to the traditional Mediterranean diet. For centuries people in countries like Italy followed a basic diet that worked very well for them. People eating the traditional Italian diet have less high cholesterol, high blood pressure, and cancer. A recent study of the people in Okinawa (an island close to Japan) found that a similar diet produced more healthy people over one hundred years old than anywhere else on this planet. For the purposes of this book, I have synthesized the best factors of all these recognized healthy diets. What do they have in common? You guessed it: *Foods that do not promote inflammation in the body.*

These nutritional strategies contain a wealth of foods that assist the immune system and the organ of blood cleansing, the liver. These diets are not loaded with heavy indigestible fats, like the trans fats found in many processed foods of the

What are the basics of the healthy traditional diet of many Oriental and Mediterranean cultures?

1. Lots of fresh fruits and vegetables, at least twice daily. Try a variety, and eat 6 to 9 cups' worth a day. Fresh is best, frozen adequate, and canned okay if there isn't too much salt or hidden sugar.

2. Small amounts of meat, less than 4 ounces per serving, and not necessarily every day. Excess meat, especially meat dense with saturated fats, is hard on the liver, kidneys, and intestines and takes a long time to fully digest. Fish several times weekly.

3. Some whole grains. Whole grains have far more fiber, vitamins, and antioxidants than the processed white-flour products. For example, oatmeal, brown rice, and whole-wheat bread, and even the rarer grains: amaranth and buckwheat. Potatoes are starchy, and to make them tasty, many believe, they have to be covered with butter or sour cream, or some other high-calorie or salty addition. All traditional diets around the world include a good source of fiber, vitamins, and complex carbohydrates. Among these are beans, peas, lentils, and chickpeas, all of them tasty and filling. Eat a variety of these as well.

4. Good-quality fats. The Mediterranean diet uses the best cooking and salad oil in the world: *olive oil.* Canola is also good. Avoid margarine, hydrogenated oils, and corn, peanut, and safflower oils. Butter in small amounts is better than margarine. Use cold-pressed virgin oil. We need to ingest healthy fats, particularly the omega-3 fatty acids.

5. Not a lot of baked or fried white-flour products. *Minimal fried foods. Minimal dairy products.** Cow's milk is better for cows. Recommended are small portions of butter, cheese, and yogurt occasionally. Be aware of the big calcium scam. Many fruits and vegetables contain adequate calcium, and people in various cultures grow healthy bones without cow's milk.

6. Minimal sugar and sugar-based foods. Excess sugar contributes to diabetes, inflammation, and a host of other problems, discussed later in this chapter.

---

*Some people might have food allergies that promote inflammation. African Americans, for example, are predisposed to milk allergies. Common foods that can cause allergies in some people include peanut butter, milk, wheat, corn, and the nightshade family (tomatoes, green peppers, and potatoes). If you suspect a food allergy, try a rotation diet where for a month you omit the suspected food. Also, see a nutritionist or a doctor familiar with nutritional medicine.

7. Healthy additions to the regular diet include various kinds of nuts and seeds (loaded with nutrients), seaweeds (high in minerals), and fermented foods like miso and yogurt. Italians and Asians use an abundance of herbs in their diet. Many of the spices and herbs reduce inflammation, assist the stomach and liver, and promote healthy immune response.

modern American diet. This diet is quite unlike the fast-food culture that dominates America and now many other countries in the world.

What is the basis of the fast-food diet? White-flour products—often loaded in hydrogenated fats, sugar, and salt—as well as greasy meat, dairy products, and puffy white food in general. This is the proinflammatory diet. This is the white-food diet, a fact that will be emphasized in this book.

FOUR NEGATIVE SUBSTANCES THAT HAVE INFILTRATED
THE AMERICAN DIET

❋ Partially hydrogenated oils in many processed foods, fried foods, processed meat, and margarine. Hydrogenation is a process used by the food industry to convert unsaturated oil into a more saturated and solid fat, a product that is less perishable. Not only are these fats hard to digest, but they interfere with cholesterol and, perhaps worst of all, interfere with the good fats. The deficiency of healthy fats in the American diet is a major theme of this book. See the discussion of good-quality fats on page 41.

❋ Sugar. Many kinds of supermarket processed foods contain hidden sugars. Some sugar is not so hidden. Pop drinks are liquid sugar. Sugar has no inherent nutrients. It is pure calories that turn to fat, overload the liver and pancreas, and create false energy. Like the previously mentioned harmful fats, excess sugar is proinflammatory. This does not mean that people cannot enjoy an occasional treat, a delicious dessert, but the amount of sugar consumed each year by each individual is phenomenal, over one hundred pounds. Sugar is moderately addictive and makes the food industry tons of money—it is now everywhere. Artificial sweeteners—are they any better? There are pros and cons, mostly cons.

❋ Chemicals from pesticide and herbicide residue in vegetables and meat; from air and water pollution. Tragically, many of our fish—one of the healthiest foods—contain increasing levels of heavy metal toxicity. Cows, chickens, and other domestic animals are fed antibiotics, steroids, and food loaded with chemical residue. Eat organic as much as possible, wash vegetables, and support organic agriculture. Read about line of defense 3, detoxification.

✳ Avoid a daily white-flour diet: for example, muffin or doughnut for breakfast, white-bread sandwich for lunch, and white pasta for dinner. Eat some complex carbohydrates: fresh vegetables, oatmeal, brown rice, bran cereal, beans, and whole-grain breads. Try protein foods for breakfast. Above all, enjoy a variety of fresh foods daily. Don't have one kind of green vegetable; there are many that are tasty and contain different nutrients. Try a variety of root vegetables: carrots, yams, parsnips, and turnips. They are rich in nutrients and satisfying.

Digestion

The basic fuel of the body is created in the digestive system. The digestive tract is hardworking and well designed. Treated with respect, it works well enough day after day, converting our food into energy and eliminating wastes. Digestion starts in the mouth with the partial breakdown of foods, and then continues in the stomach and small intestine. The churning and breakdown allow the basic nutrients to be absorbed into the walls of the small intestine: proteins, the basic building blocks of all cells; quality fats for a variety of necessary chemical functions; vitamins and minerals; and carbohydrates for basic fuel. This incredible array of nutrients then goes into the machine of our body via the cleanser—the liver—which filters out chemicals and distributes nutrients to the heart for general circulation. Nutrients in the blood then nourish all the cells of the body and the hundreds of different functions that keep the body going. The heart continues to beat, the hormones are manufactured, the lungs breathe, and the nervous system sends out thousands of messages per second. Waste products continue on their way from the small intestine into the large intestine and are then expelled.

Overlooked and abused in America is the intestinal tract. This poor organ system is under siege in America and has been since the inception of the white-food and sugar diet. At thirty feet long with a surface area the size of a small field, this tract is absolutely essential to good health. In the small intestine, food is broken down into molecules small enough to be transported to the cellular level. A key process of energy absorption takes place here, as well as an important stage of detoxification. We do not need the waste products of food and metabolism. They need to be eliminated daily; otherwise, toxification begins to creep into the whole body. The modern white-food diet, excess medical drugs like antibiotics, and emotional stress all play havoc on the beleaguered intestines. Lack of fiber creates a sluggish and lazy intestine, subject to disease and permeated with toxins that can then affect the rest of the body. Part of the immune system exists in the walls of the intestines. Antibiotics, which are overused today, kill good bacteria that have numerous health-promoting functions, including the elimination of bad bacteria! It is the firm contention of this book that health of the intestines is as important as health of the liver and immune system. Many inflammatory diseases have their root in dysfunctional intestines, including the very common irritable bowel syndromes, and even problems of the skin and immune system. Sadly, millions of Americans have poorly functioning intestines.

Treating the intestines well includes the dietary suggestions in this section. It also includes using probiotics like acidophilus for those with bowel and other problems. See appendix 2. Also, consult line of defense 3, detoxification.

To a Large Extent We Are What We Eat

Quality nutrition, the way we eat, and the process of utilization determine, to a large extent, the basic energy of the machine. When we overeat the rich, refined foods, we are loading down our digestive tract with a sometimes intolerable burden. Eat smaller meals and start with something filling and satisfying like a vegetable soup (nondairy) or some fruit and crackers.

What Is Especially Important?

We need *protein* every day for energy and muscles, but not protein laden with saturated and hydrogenated fats. Small amounts of lean beef or fish; occasional eggs; maybe cheese two or three times weekly are all possibilities. I was in a restaurant the other day enjoying one of my favorite meals: teriyaki beef with rice and salad, and a tasty microbrew. As I walked out I saw a man and a woman, both grossly overweight, consuming huge hamburgers with cheese and a monstrous pile of French fries. The man, who must have been around forty, had the huge belly of someone predisposed to diabetes, high cholesterol, or high blood pressure. This excess of protein, fats, and refined carbohydrates is the source of much needless suffering and poor-quality energy. Without doubt it is the source of metabolic syndrome, an inflammatory precursor to many diseases.

Metabolic syndrome is now recognized as a predisposition to obesity, sluggishness, and diseases like high cholesterol and diabetes. The prime cause of this common syndrome is a diet that consists primarily of refined carbohydrates and potatoes, sugar, and too much protein. This is the infamous white-food diet, a major theme of this book. Over 80 percent of heart problems and diabetes are linked to a faulty diet and lack of exercise. A healthy diet can also reduce a high percentage of cancers.

We need the vitamins and minerals found in fruits, vegetables, nuts, seeds, fish, and meat. Plants and kitchen herbs contain *phytochemicals*, valuable plant chemicals that are not vitamins or nutrients. These include carotenoids and flavonoids—numerous in vegetables, herbs, and fruits—which contain multiple healing benefits, most notably detoxifying and reducing inflammation.

Equally important for reducing inflammation are the *omega-3 fatty acids* found in some plants, seeds, and fish. Not manufactured by the body, omega-3 fatty acids are one of the foundations of abundant health. They play a major role in decreasing inflammation anywhere in the body. Furthermore, they are healthy for the heart, arteries, and brain. Deficiency of omega-3 fatty acids is implicated in heart disease, joint pain, depression, attention deficit disorder, and even in problems of brain functioning. Deficiency of these crucial healthy fats leads to premature aging and problems of cognition, most notably losing the memory. The brain, unlike muscle and bone, is over 60 percent fat, and the importance of the omega-3 fatty acids cannot be underestimated in brain health. For more information about healthy fats, consult *Fats That Heal, Fats That Kill* by Udo Erasmus.

To reiterate: There are good fats, most notably the omega-3 fatty acids, that are absolutely essential for good health and longevity. Fat-free diets or even low-fat diets can be harmful if they exclude these essential healthy fats. Ironically, studies have shown that dieters who cut out fats suffer in vain and predispose themselves to inflammatory-based diseases. The

major obstacle to weight loss is the massive amounts of refined flour and sugar products that go down the hatch daily,
hourly.

We need *carbohydrates,* but not an extensive amount,
maybe 40 percent of our daily diet. These primarily come
from grains, vegetables, and fruits. Complex carbohydrates—
vegetables, beans, oatmeal, whole-grain products, brown
rice—are more of a complete food than white-flour products,
potatoes, and white rice. For example, brown rice, which has
not been overly processed, retains valuable fiber and minerals
that white rice does not contain. Of course, this doesn't mean
we have to give up white-flour pasta or white rice but that we
need to add more of the complex carbohydrates found in vegetables and whole grains. Remember, potatoes are a bland,
starchy food that is often drenched in butter or ketchup.
French fries and other deep-fried foods might taste good, but
they are empty foods loaded with poor-quality fats. They are
a good example of what I call a devitalized food. But I do love
them once in a while, even with that ketchup (loaded with
secret sugar!).

Basic Guidelines for Daily Food

Those who have medical problems should also consult a
nutritionist or a doctor knowledgeable about foods. The diet
recommended here is not vegetarian. A vegetarian diet is

The Skinny on Processed Snack Foods

Most common snack foods found at the counters of convenience stores are loaded with refined flour, fats, and salt or sugar. Even the supposedly low-fat items and salad dressings are stocked with sugar and saturated fats. These gunk up our bodies and create inflammation. Trans fats, which can be compared to chemical sludge, are very common in margarine, snack foods, commercial salad dressings, and countless processed foods. *Beware of trans fats.* A recent addition to processed foods, trans fats are harmful. Nutritionists have been suspicious of them for thirty years. Established medicine is now raising a flag, and the FDA will soon require the food industry to label trans fats. The listing of saturated fats on a label is often a sufficient warning.

good for some people, but those who adopt this diet must research carefully how to obtain a full range of protein, vitamins, and quality fats. Some vegetarians subsist on dairy, white flour, some vegetables, and sugary items. They will not be vigorous people. Meat and eggs are highly nourishing foods, but they should not be eaten in excess. Sugar is not a poison, but it should only be used for treats and special

Good and Bad News

Yes, we need to spend more time in the kitchen to ensure our food is good quality. At restaurants, order food with discrimination and care. Stay away from fried foods (often, restaurants reuse cooking oils over and over), watch out for hidden sugars, and avoid many of the commercial salad dressings. Olive oil and vinegar with a little seasoning is an excellent salad dressing. Enjoy soups with lots of vegetables, mixed vegetable dishes, and meat with vegetables. Be wary of food with lots of cooked oil, dairy, and fried or processed meats. When you eat, eat and enjoy. Don't watch television, read the paper, or get into arguments.

occasions. A long-term high-protein diet is a strain on the liver, kidneys, and intestine: In the intestines, meat takes far longer to break down than vegetable matter.

The number-one fact is that food should be, as much as possible, fresh and whole—*real food as it exists in nature.* Eat a real apple, not bottled juice, which is high in sugars. If you eat eggs occasionally, eat real eggs from free-range chickens not loaded with drugs and not kept in tiny cages their whole lives. If you love oatmeal for breakfast, eat real oatmeal that takes a

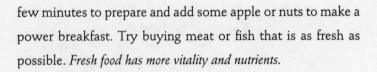

few minutes to prepare and add some apple or nuts to make a power breakfast. Try buying meat or fish that is as fresh as possible. *Fresh food has more vitality and nutrients.*

SAMPLE DIETARY PLAN

This sample plan is for those who want specific guidelines. For more detail, appendix 6 lists books and other sources.

Breakfast: For those who live in cold countries, there are several breakfasts that are recommended.

1. Oatmeal, a warming food, with low-fat milk (you can substitute soy milk), maybe with some nuts, raisins, or cut-up apple. Tea or coffee.

2. One or two eggs, maybe twice weekly, with whole-wheat toast and perhaps some beans and fruit on the side.

3. Simple on-the-go breakfast: whole-wheat toast with a little butter and fruit jam. Avoid, as much as possible, protein drinks and energy bars—highly processed foods. For those who want absorbable energizing foods, try the green food supplements, either tablets or powder. Smoothies with fruit and other goodies are excellent once in a while.

4. Yes, I am going to say it: If you like them, enjoy bacon or sausages and eggs once in a while.

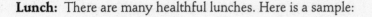

Lunch: There are many healthful lunches. Here is a sample:

1. Chicken soup with salad.

2. Turkey sandwich with pickles on the side and a salad.

3. Hearty chili or vegetable soup, with whole-wheat bread on the side with a little cheese.

4. Teriyaki chicken with mushrooms, onions, and brown rice.

Dinner: Here are examples of healthful, tasty dinners.

1. Chicken marinated for an hour in lemon, sautéed lightly in olive oil with spices for flavoring. A vegetable side dish like boiled spinach, broccoli, or carrots. Brown rice.

2. Small strips of marinated beef cooked with ginger. Mixed steamed vegetables on the side.

3. Broiled salmon with lime and pepper, with salad and vegetable soup.

4. Pot roast: beef cooked with carrots, onions, and other vegetables.

5. Vegetarian chili with tortillas and salsa, a little grated cheese, lettuce, and tomatoes. Or add a small amount of ground beef, turkey, or chicken to the beans. Remember, beans, peas, and lentils are not only filling and satisfying, they are very healthy, a good source of protein, healthy oils, and vitamin E.

Desserts: Fruit, rice pudding, and oatmeal cookies are a few examples, preferably light on the sugar and hydrogenated fats. Once in a while enjoy a slice of cheesecake or chocolate ice cream, or raspberries and cream. When I was in France, I enjoyed the best desserts in the world at dinner for a whole week!

Liquids: Water, green tea, other herbal teas like chamomile, black tea, coffee, soy milk, rice milk, occasional fruit juices (better to eat the whole fruit). Wine and beer, in moderation. Wine is loaded with antioxidants. Also, it is best not to drink too many caffeinated beverages a day. For example, for many people, more than three cups of coffee can be excessive. Personally I love black tea and coffee, one or two cups daily. Yes, I confess I sometimes add a little sugar and cream to my coffee at Sunday-morning breakfast.

Great News: The Bottom Line in Relation to Daily Diet

The guidelines given are a good foundation for better health and energy, but experience shows that one cannot restrict Americans when it comes to enjoying the "naughty" foods. We should enjoy the treats and "sinful" foods, perhaps not every day, but several times weekly. Fatty foods like bacon, chocolate, barbecued ribs, and ice cream are just plain delicious and irresistible. I love all these items. Sunday breakfast at an inn in Vermont can be a downright orgy of fatty foods: cream and coffee, bacon and eggs, and pancakes with butter. As long as we follow the basic guidelines—and we don't have any medical restrictions—we can enjoy these treats several times a week. The fresh vegetables and fruits, the foods rich in antioxidants and omega-3 fatty acids, will offset the potentially harmful quality of the rich treats. Some of the foods in the next section are particularly protective and energizing.

Super Foods

Some foods are particularly good for cleansing and energizing. These are emphasized in this general program to defend our health. Why do I call them "super foods"? Because they have multiple healing benefits: They inhibit germs, boost the immune system, and support the liver and intestines. You guessed it. They are anti-inflammatory. These include:

* Garlic, multiple healing benefits like thinning the blood and inhibiting nasty germs.
* Mushrooms support the immune system and thin the blood. Try a variety of mushrooms. They can be added to countless casseroles, soups, salads, and meat courses.
* For snacks, try cantaloupe and watermelon, high in vitamins A and C as well as therapeutic phytochemicals.

✳ Olive oil—omega-9 fatty acids, similar to omega-3. Cold-pressed olive oil is the best kitchen oil for us to consume.

✳ Leafy greens—rich in fiber, vitamins, and antioxidants. One should eat a bowl of fresh or cooked greens every day. Iceberg lettuce is a bogus green. Try romaine, Boston lettuce, kale, collards, watercress, and mustard greens.

✳ Herbs like parsley, sage, rosemary, and thyme—yes, I said it! For example, rosemary is good for the brain and contains antioxidants that protect the liver and inhibit formation of cancer cells. Liberally, enjoy herbs and spices every day.

✳ Berries. Raspberries and blueberries are common favorites, loaded with vitamins and antioxidants. Tufts University research has found that blueberries are abundantly loaded with antioxidants.

✳ Acidophilus, found in fermented food like yogurt (buy real yogurt without sugar and preservatives!), miso, and pickles.

✳ Salmon, cod, and mackerel: truly super foods, especially the wild salmon. Farm-raised salmon is not as healthy as the wild Alaska salmon.

✳ Beef raised on the range with grass. Try buying free-range beef and chicken not raised with antibiotics and steroids, and not fed the staple of agribusiness farms: corn. Corn-raised beef is more inflammatory than grass-fed. Cows have grazed on grass for centuries, until the modern American era—the era of fast food and agribusiness.

✳ Lots of root vegetables like carrots, yams, and parsnips. These are loaded with antioxidants and vitamins, as well as a variety of healthy fibers.

Save the Health of Our Children

Promote healthy nutrition with kids. Many health problems will be avoided. Kids start off their lives inundated with propaganda from the sugary fast-food industry. It is hard to break the habit of greasy, sugary white foods once they have started. "Oh, I hate vegetables." This is the cry heard too frequently by frustrated parents. It is a fact that children raised without poor-quality fats and sugar are healthier, less prone to colds, earaches, digestive problems, hyperactivity, and a host of other problems in America's youth. If children follow the above guidelines, they will be healthier and happier. They do not begin their adulthood with the subtle inflammation syndrome. Tragic to say, but American fast-food culture is being exported around the world faster than you can say McDonald's. This proinflammatory diet, high in bad fats and refined sugar, is tragically low in omega-3 fatty acids that are necessary for a healthy emotional life and brain functions. The result, a steadily rising index of inflammatory diseases: high cholesterol, heart attacks, diabetes, obesity, and numerous bowel diseases—not too mention rapid mood swings.

Meat Controversy

Americans eat too much meat, especially meat that is rich in saturated fats: luncheon meats, hot dogs, fried meats, and fatty cuts. *Six hundred million* Big Macs and twenty billion hot dogs are consumed yearly. Sadly, there is a suspicion that excess fatty meat can lead to some kinds of cancer, not to mention a variety of bowel diseases. Chicken, lean beef, pork, turkey, and game meats are excellent sources of tasty protein. Some people prefer organic meats, a tendency that might prove more and more popular as confidence in the safety of beef is eroded.

Eating According to Body Type

This section is not meant to be a specific guide about what kind of diet you should follow. It is offered as an example that our daily diet needs to be a little different according to our body type. People have needs for different kinds of fuel, and some have a weakness for certain kinds of cheap fuel.

If you look around a busy city street you will see all kinds of body types. People are different. Some are tall and thin, others short and pudgy—with everyone else in between. Oriental medicine has a way of simplifying this array of types: the five basic constitutional types. Each of these five types is a generic description. These different types are different not only in form but also in activity, temperament, and energy. They can have different nutritional needs and sometimes need to moderate their diets according to their type.

EARTH TYPE: The stereotype is the happy bon vivant like the rotund, jolly Falstaff in Shakespeare's plays. Energy centers on the stomach and pancreas. Health problems tend to gravitate around digestion and metabolism: diabetes, hypothyroidism, obesity, and stomach problems. The earth type tends to be phlegmatic and earthy and is prone to weight problems. They often love food and the simple pleasures of life and can have a good fund of energy. In work they tend to be practical, hard-working, and reliable. Major dietary weaknesses are sugar, sweets, and carbohydrates. They love big bowls of pasta with tomato sauce. For more energy they need to consume less carbohydrates, more vegetables, and quality protein—and little sugar; they get addicted to it. It is important to emphasize that being a little plump or chubby, whatever the expression, is not a negative thing—often an expression of body type.

AIR TYPE: The stereotypical air type is thin, wiry, and active, though sometimes thin and delicate. The thoughtful, sensitive artist like Marc Chagall is a good representative of this type. Health problems center around the lungs and breathing, and they are prone to asthma, sinus problems, and colds. They can eat sparingly, often snack-type foods, and need to adopt a balanced diet. They often overindulge in spicy foods or stimulants like coffee. They need to consume more fish, lean meat, omega-3 fatty acids, and root vegetables like yams and carrots.

WATER TYPE: This is the well-known kidney type who is often intense and preoccupied, and when in ill health tends to bladder problems, fatigue, or anxiety. The stereotypical water type is John F. Kennedy, who had a host of health problems and pain under his charming exterior. This kind can eat haphazardly, veering to extremes: too much caffeine, fats, or protein. They need to add a variety of fruits and complex carbohydrates to their diet, decrease chemicals and alcohol, and eat foods that are nourishing and grounding: fish, root vegetables, leafy greens, and seeds.

WOOD TYPE: The active athlete or the competitive businessman who runs every morning before his commute. The wood type can be tall and muscular, or too lean and hyperactive. Michael Jordan, the basketball star, is a good representative of this type. Each type has an excess trajectory in habits, temperament, and foods. The wood type can be overcompetitive, a perfectionist who cannot stand the more plodding style of the earth type. They tend to stimulants like caffeine, excess protein, and fats and often benefit from a more vegetarian diet. They overtax their livers with meat, alcohol, and cigarettes. More than other types, the wood type tends to stomach troubles, blood pressure problems, and high cholesterol. They can do with some guidance about stress reduction.

FIRE TYPE: The stereotypical fire type is active and enthusiastic, the life of the party, the chatty person in the office. While they tend to be small and lean, fire types can come in different sizes and shapes. Often they exhibit reddish color, pink cheeks, reddish ears, and other signs of the "fire." In disharmony they tend to be impatient, anxious, and too zealous. They love fiery foods: spices, chili peppers, coffee, and alcohol. They can binge on fatty foods and then drink coffee and snacks for a few days. They need to consume more cooling, grounding foods to stabilize their wayward energies, to decrease the fried foods, coffee, sugar, and other stimulants. Particularly good for this kind is fish, greens, root vegetables, and whole grains. A fish, bean, or turkey soup with vegetables could be one of their staples.

Once people begin a nutritional program that fits their body type, they can look to other solutions to defend their health and promote good energy.

SOLUTIONS TO ENERGY DEFICIENCY AND LACK OF STAMINA

❋ Get adequate exercise, moderate and daily, perhaps half an hour. One of the several benefits to exercise is that it stimulates deep breathing.

❋ Reduce excess stress—see line of defense 2.

❋ Detoxify and reduce inflammation—see lines of defense 3 and 4.

❋ Be aware of underlying diseases like underactive thyroid, which governs how we burn our food. See your doctor for persistent fatigue, especially when accompanied by temperature changes, changes in mood, any persistent internal pain, or headaches.

❋ Keep the intestines healthy so wastes and toxins do not accumulate in the body. Americans do not eat enough fiber or drink enough water. Helpful bacteria, which live in the intestines, keep harmful bacteria in check. These positive bacteria also help the body to synthesize valuable nutrients. When using antibiotics, supplement with probiotics like acidophilus. Modern diet and medications play havoc on the bowels, resulting in digestive diseases, inflammation, and poor energy. This includes abuse of antibiotics, excess sugar, anti-

Energy Herbs

Herbs are whole-food medicines that contain a variety of nutrients that support the body and its functions. Adaptogens are a kind of herbal medicine that is particularly good for busy, stressed people. A classic adaptogen is Siberian ginseng, which supports the body when tired or stressed out. Herbal medicines are kind to the body, not abusive like some medical drugs. They do not tax the immune system, intestines, or liver. See appendices 2 and 3 for more information on therapeutic herbs for energy.

inflammatory drugs, and steroidal drugs. Fermented foods like yogurt, sauerkraut, and miso support the healthy bacteria, but make sure that when you purchase these items that they are real foods, not loaded with chemicals or sugar. Many commercial yogurts are not so healthy. Consult appendix 2.

✳ Give the body a boost with food supplements like green food powder, vitamins, and herbal and green tea.

✳ Take herbs for energy, including Siberian ginseng, Asian ginseng, and ashwagandha. Note: There are restrictions on herbal medicines for pregnant or nursing women and those who are on some kind of long-term medication. Also, ginseng should not be used by those who are young and healthy, hyperactive, or suffering from high blood pressure. Typical dose: as recommended on label for several weeks.

✳ When the body is not working well, always consider having a medical checkup.

SUMMING UP

Food is our basic fuel for our incredible energy machine. Feed it well. Try to prepare simple healthy meals for yourself every day, and sit down and enjoy—take the time. Do not rely on fast food for energy. In time you will pay the price. Read labels. Question. Examine books with good solid information. For some excellent books on healthy food, see the selected bibliography at the end of this book. Relax when eating, and don't feel guilty for those occasional pleasures of good cuisine.

LINE OF DEFENSE 2: STRESS REDUCTION

How excess stress depletes the body and promotes inflammation and disease was discussed in chapter 2. To briefly review, excess stress creates toxins in the body, unnecessary tension, and wear and tear that can lead to disease and premature aging. Prolonged stresses in the body are one major root of many diseases, including susceptibility to harmful germs.

SOLUTIONS TO EXCESS STRESS

✳ Since one of the major stresses on the body is the modern fast-food diet, see line of defense 1.

✳ Other stresses include chemicals and inflammation; see lines of defense 2 and especially 3.

✳ Exercise is a good solution to excess stress. Several times weekly, preferably a variety of exercises, whatever appeals to you. Maybe walking briskly for half an hour three times a week and then two visits to the gym the same week. Basketball, skating, martial arts, dance, and aerobics are fine ways to let off steam, detoxify, and allow the body some fun movement. Other suggestions include tai chi, yoga, golf, and swimming.

✳ Seek help from friends or professionals during stressful times.

✳ Relaxation, fun, and play are incredibly important. Spend time every week with kids, or playing some game you like.

✳ Exercises for the heart and soul. These are very important and include singing, prayer, and meditation, as well as reading sacred books. It is a well-known fact that positive attitudes and activities have a profound effect on health.

✳ Laughter. Not much to say here.

✳ If you get sick, it is not your fault. Many illnesses are a part of the life process and cannot be avoided. When sick, turn to friends, good books, and one or several of the above-mentioned spiritual exercises. There are countless stories about people who have overcome sickness to learn profound new understandings.

✳ Certain foods and herbs can help the body adapt to stress better. See line of defense 1 and consult appendices 2 and 3.

LINE OF DEFENSE 3: DETOXIFICATION

Detoxification of the body reduces unnecessary chemical stress on the body, which is good for overall energy as well as the immune system. As was said, a hectic modern lifestyle, diet, and stress lead to toxic overload of the liver, intestines, and other organs. Multiple stresses included synthetic chemicals from drugs and pollution, chemicals created by the stress response, unhealthy saturated fats, free radicals, and excess sugar. This toxic overload, while not a disease, leads to poor-quality energy and chronic inflammatory diseases. Of course, this can take years to develop. Signs include fatigue, poor concentration, pains and aches, muscular tension, irritability, poor sleep, and swollen glands. Sadly, the groundwork for more serious diseases is firmly established. And ironically, the patient requires more painkillers and anti-inflammatory drugs, which can in the long run aggravate the whole situation. These drugs do not treat the source of the inflammation and pain. Furthermore, they overtax the liver, the main organ of detoxification; they harm the stomach; and the final paradox, they can even harm connective tissue, tendons, and ligaments—the very reason people pop them so avidly.

Americans spend billions of dollars a year on over-the-counter anti-inflammatory drugs. Each year, doctors write millions of prescriptions for pharmaceutical pain-killers. Each year, another drug is removed from the market.

The final insult to the poor body has already been mentioned several times in this book. Prolonged toxification leads to inflammation, and inflammation can confuse the immune system and make the body more susceptible to allergens, cancer cells, viruses, and bacteria. Why is it that some people never get a cold or flu in the office, even when they have not had the flu shot? Their body is balanced and healthy, the liver and immune system are working well, and the resistance is excellent. Of course, they breathe in the same virus germs. Their immune system takes care of the intrusion.

Solutions to assist toxification

❋ *Diet and nutrition.* See line of defense 1. To summarize: Eat foods rich in vitamins, antioxidants, fiber, and healthy fats. A major insult to the body in the modern world is the recent flood of harmful fats from processed foods. In the past fifty years, the food industry has inundated the market with poor-quality fats, particularly partially hydrogenated fats and trans fats, in many cooking oils, salad oils, and margarine. Reduce junk and processed foods, reduce excess sugar—it will turn to fat. Eat real food, whole food, fresh food. Drink adequate amounts of fluid each day, preferably water, black teas, or herbal teas.

❋ *Moderate fasts can assist in detoxification.* Once a month, eat lightly for a week or even three days: water, one-half cup of real lemon juice daily, apples and other fruits, vegetables, and maybe some fish. No dairy, meat, or fatty foods. Give the body a break and tune-up. If you have a medical problem, consult with your doctor before any moderate fasting. Extreme fasts—not eating at all—are not recommended without professional guidance.

❋ *Exercise moderately three to five times weekly,* twenty to thirty minutes or more. Include stretching every day for five to ten minutes. Taking time to breathe deeply is essential to good health.

✳ *Specific herbal medicines assist the liver and detoxification.* These include green tea, milk thistle, schisandra, dandelion root, and red clover. Detoxifying herbs include basil, turmeric, and rosemary. See appendices 2 and 3.

✳ *Constipation is not healthy for the bowels, liver, or whole body.* If you are not having a bowel movement every day, try more fiber foods, reduce white flour, eat a bowl of stewed prunes, oatmeal, peas, apples, and green leafy vegetables. Drink more water. Psyllium seeds are a source of plant fiber. Drink them with plenty of water. Follow directions carefully or ask your doctor. Flaxseeds are another excellent source of fiber. Senna is an herb that moves the bowels. Exercise and stretch. Always consult your doctor when experiencing any chronic bowel problems with pain, bleeding, or swelling. The health of the bowels is intimately connected to the health of the whole body and is as important as the health of the liver and immune system (see line of defense 1, under digestion). Probiotics—good bacteria—are essential for bowel health. Acidophilus found in yogurt (and some fermented food like sauerkraut) or food supplements is an example. Many modern drugs play havoc on bowel health, particularly excess antibiotics, anti-inflammatories, and steroids. What is good for the intestines? The foundation is a sensible whole-food diet with lots of onions, leeks, mushrooms, asparagus, artichoke, banana, chicory root, whole grains, all rich in substances that nourish the intestines—also called prebiotics (fructo-oligosaccharides). The intestines are sensitive to emotional and mental stress, particularly worry, fear, and anger (see line of defense 2). Sluggish bowels are too common in America—the main culprit, white-food diet.

❋ *Sweating helps the body detoxify.* The skin is an organ of elimination. Saunas, sweaty exercise like aerobics, and any other pleasurable physical activity, such as basketball, volleyball, gymnastics, skating, and brisk walking.

❋ *Take baths with lavender or rosemary powders,* and soak for at least fifteen minutes.

❋ *Massage or acupuncture.*

❋ *Calm the mind and emotions* with meditation, prayer, walking, love, and all of the above—whatever works for you.

LINE OF DEFENSE 4:
DECREASING INFLAMMATION

Inflammation is an insidious factor in many diseases. Toxification (see previous section), stress, and overuse lead to various kinds of inflammation. Basically, inflammation is a process that can be compared to the engine of a car overheating. In the body it creates heat, pain, swelling, and toxins. Everyone is familiar with the kind of inflammation when we cut our finger or sprain our ankle. In this instance, inflammation is largely a healing response by the body. For the purpose of this book, we are not so concerned about this kind of inflammation. We are concerned with subtle internal inflammation that causes disease, pain, and imbalances in the body.

Some diseases are marked by inflammation: for example, colitis, migraine headaches, sore throats, bronchitis, asthma, and most kinds of arthritis. Less well known is the low-grade systemic (whole-body) inflammation. Hard to detect, hidden, and harmful, generalized inflammation is now rampant in American society. This kind of inflammation is not a disease per se. Doctors, unless trained in holistic nutrition, know little about this disease predisposition. While generalized inflammation is not readily understood or diagnosed, there is one inexpensive and easy test, CRP. C-reactive protein can determine levels of inflammation in the body. High CRP ratings occur in people with cancer, arthritis, colitis, and infections. This subject is the source of intensive research, and in the next few years most Americans will have learned about the dangers of inflammatory syndrome. Soon other tests will be available.

Billions of dollars' worth of anti-inflammatory drugs are used each year. Untold suffering and pain result from inflammatory diseases. Tragically, the drugs do not get to the root of the problem and can, in the long run, make things worse. If inflammation goes on for too long, serious diseases are more likely: ulcerative colitis, some kinds of cancer, arthritis, Alzheimer's disease, and many others.

Inflammation is often connected to a chronic acidic condition in the body, mostly from white-food, sugary diet, excess citrus and tomato products, and excess red meat.

Inflammation is often linked to toxicity, the subject of the previous section. While its presence is often hard to detect, symptoms can raise red flags—fatigue, aches and pains, irregular bowel movements, gum problems, irritability, muscular tension, headaches, back pain, and a host of other problems. Chronic inflammation will cause pain and destroy connective tissue, leading to degeneration of joints and organs.

SOLUTIONS TO INFLAMMATION

❋ See diet and nutrition in line of defense 1. This solution is important because inflammation is often caused by pro-inflammatory foods. The foods that promote inflammation must be reduced, and foods that promote healing of inflammation should be eaten every day.

❋ Exercise—even gentle exercise—some sweating, and stretching can help the body cleanse itself. Please consult line of defense 3.

❋ Herbal remedies are well known for their ability to decrease inflammation without the side effects of pharmaceutical drugs. For those on medications or with a chronic disease, see a health

Not All Herbal Medicines and Vitamins Are Equal

Vitamin C is extraordinarily valuable, but better taken with its natural allies, the antioxidants—bioflavonoids. Selenium, a trace mineral with antioxidant properties, may prevent cancer. Many herbal remedies contain valuable antioxidants as well as properties that support the liver and decrease inflammation. Extremely important are fruits and vegetables, as well as the previously mentioned omega-3 fatty acids found in fish and some plants. Green food supplements like spirulina and blue-green algae are rich in antioxidants and other valuable nutrients.

professional for specific advice. Some herbal medicines that help decrease inflammation include red clover tea, green tea, and the herbs boswellia, turmeric, milk thistle, and schisandra. Specialized formulas are also available. See appendix 3.

❋ Antioxidants, vitamins, and supplements are excellent solutions. Vitamin E is an important antioxidant with anti-inflammatory properties. Unfortunately, not all vitamin E on the market is the same quality. Purchase the natural form of vitamin E, which is easier for the body to absorb. Natural vitamin E uses the designation d, as in d-alpha tocopherol. Syn-

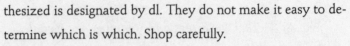

thesized is designated by dl. They do not make it easy to determine which is which. Shop carefully.

❋ Stress-reduction strategies: music, meditation, exercise, baths with herbal tonic, and many more. See line of defense 2.

SUMMING UP

In America, the common insult to the poor body has already been mentioned several times in this book. Overtaxed liver and intestines, inflammation, and weakened immune system are the groundwork for many diseases.

Prolonged toxification leads to inflammation, and inflammation can confuse the immune system and make the body more susceptible to allergens, cancer cells, viruses, and bacteria. Why is it that some people rarely get sick? One reason is that their body adapts well to multiple stresses and potential toxins, decreasing the opportunity for inflammation and disease. One major source of protection is the immune system.

LINE OF DEFENSE 5: THE IMMUNE SYSTEM, OUR MAIN SHIELD AGAINST DISEASE AGENTS

Our primary shield against invading disease agents, including bacteria, viruses, and cancer, is the immune system. We live in a sea of life, all in motion. In this sea of life are millions of bacteria and virus, many harmless, a few that can cause disease. Within the body are numerous bacteria and viruses, all kept in check by the immune system. Around the shield of our skin are countless toxins and microbes, some potential enemies. Most often, they enter through the mouth or nose, or accompany the food we eat. When we breathe in a foreign invader, say a nasty cold virus, our body's defenses marshal an attack. Our main defense against these tiny foreign "terrorists" is the immune system. The immune system is a vastly complicated and intelligent defense system. In one body, there are millions of immune cells. This is not the place to explore the intricacies of the immune system, but several facts are helpful for understanding the value of natural medicines.

There are several ways the immune system eliminates foreign invaders. The immune system creates antibodies that recognize a specific invader and then disable it. B-cells produce the antibodies. T-cells coordinate immune defenses and kill enemy cells. Part of this intricate warfare is chemical. T-cells, for example, secrete potent chemicals—lymphokines— that poison foreign invaders as well as cancer cells. The immune system is like an army with different weapons. Phagocytes, another potent weapon, gobble up foreign invaders, including viruses and harmful bacteria. Most often the flu or cold virus (or any other potentially harmful invader) is soon eliminated by the immune system, and the body then resumes health. Sometimes, the immune system is overwhelmed or just plain weak.

What hinders the immune system?

✳ Faulty diet. Consult lines of defense 1 and 2. The white, sugary, high–saturated fat diet of many Americans is not conducive to a healthy immune response.

✳ Poor bowel function can indirectly inhibit immune response. Chronic constipation leads to toxicity and inflammation.

✳ Prolonged and multiple stresses (see line of defense 2).

What helps the immune system?

✳ See line of defense 1, energy and stamina.

✳ Herbal medicines like astragalus and certain mushrooms (like maitake) can boost the immune response (see appendices 2 and 3).

✳ Positive, creative emotions and attitudes have a profound effect on the immune system (see line of defense 2).

Herbal Allies for the Immune System

Recently it has been discovered that specific foods can support the immune system—many vegetables and herbs. Some medicinal herbs are particularly rich in constituents that boost the immune system. Common ones include echinacea, astragalus, and rosemary. Astragalus, a well-known Asian plant medicine, makes the T-cells, valuable immune components, more aggressive. It also seems to stimulate other immune factors, including the natural killer cells. Astragalus is a very safe herb, with little or no side effects. Echinacea, another well-known herb, also supports immune factors and increases resistant to harmful disease agents.

Some herbs can support the immune system by inhibiting the activity of disease-causing agents. For example, the Asian herb andrographis decreases the proliferation of cancer cells by inhibiting enzymes that stimulate carcinogenesis. Each year we are discovering more about the specific healing properties of herbs (please consult appendix 3 for more information).

SUMMING UP

The body is incredibly intelligent, having evolved for millions of years to live and survive. The foods and herbs have evolved in tandem with humans and contain information that is very useful for our health. Many of the foods and herbs are like minicomputer programs that enter the vast web of the body to assist and support its life-preserving functions. By assisting the liver and immune system, natural medicines and foods are admirably suited to protect us from disease agents so rampant in our modern society. While modern drugs can target specific disease agents, when they are abused they can also overwhelm the body. Natural medicines are designed to safely assist the body's vitality and defenses.

The five lines of defense are a comprehensive strategy to maintain vigor and health. While all of them are equally important and interrelated, one or two might be more pertinent to each individual. The following chapter offers more specific guidelines for those suffering from health problems and diseases.

CHAPTER 4

Common Health Problems Related to Stress and Inflammation

THIS CHAPTER OFFERS GENERAL GUIDELINES ABOUT WHAT TO do for specific health problems. This section is not meant to be an exhaustive guideline for the wide spectrum of diseases and is not meant to be a step-by-step treatment protocol. The primary focus is how to protect the body from chemicals, disease agents, and the stresses of modern life. For example, there are foods that support the immune system and those that increase energy in times of stress. Emphasized are areas of the body that are particularly susceptible to toxins and pollutants. For example, environmental pollution and other threats often affect the lungs, breathing, and sinuses, as well as the skin, eyes, and liver. These areas and functions will be addressed. Equally important are those methods that promote health, energy, and disease resistance.

Under each heading is a brief discussion of the problem. The five defenses, discussed in chapter 3, are frequently referred to under each heading. When consulting the following sections, please remember:

❋ Do not stop taking medications without medical advice, and for those who are using prescription drugs, please consult a physician before making any drastic changes in diet or supplements.

❋ Some herbal medicines are suggested in this book. Consult your doctor if you plan to use an herbal remedy for medicinal purposes while taking a prescription drug. Consult appendices 2 and 3 for more advice about herbal medicines.

❋ If you suspect a food allergy, see an appropriate health professional. Some people are allergic to wheat, dairy, and other foods, but they do not know it.

The suggestions in this chapter are not meant to replace the good and necessary care of doctors and are not intended for serious and chronic diseases. For medical advice on diet or herbal medicines, people should seek professional advice.

There are many symptoms that should send us to the

proper health care provider. These include high fever, any prolonged or severe bleeding, unusual changes in stools, any unusual lumps or bumps, difficulty breathing, severe headaches, head or eye injury, relentless vomiting and cramping, and sharp recurring pains.

The basis of natural and holistic medicine is a healthy terrain and a robust constitution. Consult a professional when you must, and be humble in the face of the great mystery of disease and health. Often healing comes from places we don't expect. It might involve patching up a family relationship or changing careers rather than taking a drug or natural remedy, or it could involve antibiotics and surgery, or it might be best served by prayer and meditation. So use your common sense, consult the professionals when necessary, learn more than you can, and enjoy the great bounty of Mother Nature.

A Note on Dosages for Herbal Medicines and Vitamins

Specific dosage information is difficult to offer because people are individuals with their own needs, which vary depending on age, weight, sex, and other factors. There are, however, several useful guidelines. Those who are using herbal medicines or vitamins for medical reasons should always consult a trained health professional; this is especially true for those using medical drugs daily. Otherwise, vitamins and herbal medicines can be taken according to the labels. Common sense can prevail here: For example, most multivitamins (the most common vitamin supplement) are taken once or twice daily. Vitamin C can be taken for several days or even weeks in doses of 500 to 1,000 mg daily.

The term "herbal medicine" refers to professional-quality herbs that are found as tablets, capsules, or liquid, and which are purchased at pharmacies or health food stores. Instructions about how to take these natural medicines are found on the labels. Herbal medicines can be found as single herbs or in formulas. Someone might, for example, purchase echinacea tablets for cold prevention, and read that two tablets should be taken daily for a few days. Most often these herbal medicines are taken for the short term. Herbal formulas are a blend of herbs that work well together. These are also called "synergistic herbal formulas." Oriental herbal medicine makes extensive and intelligent use of hundreds of herbal formulas, many of which have been used for hundreds of years. They have a safe and remarkable track record. These formulas exist for a wide range of health problems, but perhaps the best use is for health promotion. For example, the famous herbal medicine astragalus, which boosts the immune system, is found in several herbal formulas for fatigue, weak immune system, and prevention of colds. Astragalus is then complemented and enhanced by the inclusion of the other herbs, making for a more potent natural medicine.

Herbal teas are less concentrated home remedies that can be brewed in the kitchen. When making teas for health reasons, I prefer to brew two bags of a specific tea (for example, peppermint for stomachache) in hot water for at least five minutes. Otherwise the tea can be too weak.

To review: Herbal medicines can be purchased as tablets, capsules, and liquids, either as the single herb or in a time-honored formula. The generic dosage is given on the label but can be changed according to the needs of the patient or the advice of a physician. Also consult appendix 3, Medicinal Plants, and my book *Power Herbs*.

Conditions and Suggested Solutions

Acne: See Skin.

Adrenal Exhaustion: See Fatigue and Exhaustion.

Aging: See Longevity.

Alcoholism: An insidious and harmful addiction that should be addressed with counseling and psychological support. See lines of defense 2 and 3. It is a good idea to seek out professional advice about diet, detoxification, and medicinal herbs, which can be most helpful in this condition. In Oriental medicine, treatment of the liver and nervous system is

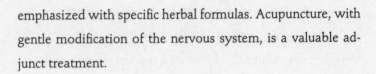

emphasized with specific herbal formulas. Acupuncture, with gentle modification of the nervous system, is a valuable adjunct treatment.

Allergies: We can define an allergy as an inappropriate response by the body's immune system to a substance that is not normally harmful. Over-response by the immune system can be a factor in some very troubling diseases, including asthma, rheumatoid arthritis, and eczema. Conventional medicine is very puzzled by the cause of many such diseases. It is the hypothesis of this book that generalized inflammation is a background in all these diseases. The contained or generalized inflammation—for example, in the lungs—confuses the immune cells and, after a while, they begin to attack the body's own cells. It is a known fact that inflammation—as in heart disease or asthma—creates a constriction that leads to distressing and even life-threatening symptoms.

Most often we consider allergies a reaction by the immune system to a foreign substance: dust, pollen, or other airborne products. Common symptoms include sneezing, nasal congestion, itchy eyes, coughing, and sore throat. Hay fever is an allergic reaction to pollen, most commonly in spring. Why is it that some people get hay fever, while some could swim in the pollen and not suffer one sneeze? Conventional wisdom might say that the hay fever sufferer inherited the genes from one or both parents. There could be truth to this, but how is it that people can rid themselves of hay fever without shots or drugs? They do it by eliminating factors—notably inflammation—that predispose the immune system to over-react. I have seen many people rid themselves of troubling allergies by improving their diet, supporting their liver, and reducing toxification in the body. One reaches to the root of allergy, and the symptoms can diminish dramatically. Long-term use of allergy medication can produce side effects.

For a general overview about possible solutions to allergies, refer to lines of defense 1, 3, and 5. For more detailed advice regarding stubborn allergies, see a holistic health professional knowledgeable about nutritional medicine.

For those who don't want to take pharmaceutical drugs, there are some herbal medicines, like nettle leaf capsules, eyebright, and elderberry, that can relieve symptoms. Quercetin is a plant constituent that can also be helpful, as can vitamin C with flavonoids. Nasalcromyn—an over-the-counter allergy medication—is a synthetic version of a natural plant constituent, a bioflavonoid.

Some allergies are aggravated by foods: for example, wheat, dairy, or corn. Try a rotation diet or see the appropriate health professional.

Some allergies stem from poor assimilation of foods from the small intestines. Because of chronic bowel inflammation and faulty diet, the body is flooded with toxins, which then overload the immune system. See Leaky Gut Syndrome later in this chapter.

Finally, the glut of allergies in America is largely aggravated by the white-food diet of many Americans. White flour, sugar, and saturated fats clog up the body and compromise the liver and immune system. Some people refer to the mucus-forming diet, the fast-food diet that creates lots of mucus and phlegm. For more information, consult the following headings in this chapter: Leaky Gut Syndrome, Immune System, and Sinusitis.

Alzheimer's Disease: This is a common kind of dementia, marked by memory loss, confusion, and mood swings. Alzheimer's, a degenerative disorder that damages brain cells, can take years to manifest and progress. It is a serious and complex problem that requires professional advice. However, some researchers believe that underlying inflammation is a factor that can produce Alzheimer's. See lines of defense 3 and 4. Degeneration, a feature in many chronic and elderly diseases, is often a flag that indicates toxification, leading to prolonged and damaging inflammation. There is also some indication that heavy metal toxicity (aluminum and mercury) could result in some cases of Alzheimer's. Hereditary factors must also be taken into account, as well as long-term nutritional deficiencies, particularly an excess of proinflammatory fats and a deficiency in healthy omega-3 fatty acids.

If seeking natural medicines for this condition, consult an appropriate health professional. Herbal medicines can offer some assistance to these patients, including ginkgo, bacopa, and omega-3 supplements. Consult remedies under Memory. Acupuncture, herbal medicine, and nutritional solutions are highly recommended as positive adjunct treatment.

Angina: Essentially, angina is a muscle cramp in the heart muscle. The heart never rests, and sometimes it cannot receive the oxygen it needs for this constant work. Symptoms include tightness and discomfort in the chest, including sharp pains. There are several excellent pharmaceutical drugs for angina, and this condition always requires expert medical attention. Healthy foods, herbal medicines, and moderate exercise have a major role in the prevention of this condition. The health of the heart is dependent on the health of the blood vessels: The blood vessels can be afflicted by poor-quality fats, free radicals, and other biochemical insults resulting from toxification and inflammation. Please consult lines of defense 1, 2, 3, and 4.

For prevention of angina and other heart problems,

consume foods that thin the blood, like mushrooms, onions, and garlic, and stay away from the proinflammatory foods, particularly the poor-quality fats in hydrogenated oils, margarine, many vegetable oils, and fried foods. A variety of vegetables is recommended, particularly the dark leafy green vegetables.

There are several natural supplements that have been shown to be particularly healthy for the heart: These include carnitine, magnesium, coenzyme Q_{10}, vitamin E, and the herb hawthorn. Consult with your physician. A typical dose of hawthorn would be two capsules twice daily, 160 mg.

Anti-inflammatory Solutions: As has been said, internal inflammation is a factor in many diseases and a cause of much pain. We do not need to depend on medications that mask the pain and inflammation. We can moderate the all too common inflammatory responses in the body. Consult lines of defense 1, 2, 3, and 4. Also, consult Cleansing in this chapter.

Many foods can promote inflammation. Other foods can moderate inflammation. This important fact has already been discussed in chapter 3. Some herbs with anti-inflammatory properties include bupleurum, burdock, echinacea, garlic, goldenseal, licorice, rosemary, turmeric, oregano, and yellow dock. Herbal medicines that reduce inflammation are different from the pharmaceutical drugs; they reduce the underlying cause of inflammation without the potential harm to the body. Quercetin and bromelain are natural anti-inflammatories. Omega-3 fatty acids can be an important supplement, as well as vitamin E. These natural supplements can reduce inflammation and prolong a healthy life.

Does this book promote the complete avoidance of pharmaceutical nonsteroidal anti-inflammatory drugs (NSAIDs)? Of course not. They can be useful and necessary, but mostly for the short term. Side effects and dangers come from long-term use—weeks and months.

Anxiety and Nervousness: For simple everyday anxiety and nervousness that do not require medical attention, consult line of defense 2. For a good home remedy for minor stress and nervousness, try strong cups of Saint-John's-wort tea. The fresh dried flower tops are a good remedy for most in times of stress and overwork. Saint-John's-wort is not just a remedy for those who are depressed. Used as a tea, it is a good all-around remedy.

For more advice, please consult Stress later in this chapter, as well as Sleeplessness.

Arthritis: Joint pain. Anyone suffering from painful joints should be cognizant of the fact that there are multiple solutions, including an initial medical checkup, diet, exercise, and

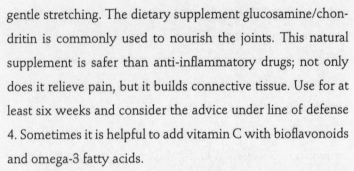

gentle stretching. The dietary supplement glucosamine/chondritin is commonly used to nourish the joints. This natural supplement is safer than anti-inflammatory drugs; not only does it relieve pain, but it builds connective tissue. Use for at least six weeks and consider the advice under line of defense 4. Sometimes it is helpful to add vitamin C with bioflavonoids and omega-3 fatty acids.

For stubborn cases of arthritis, I suggest dietary changes as well as massage and acupuncture. Helpful herbal remedies include black cohosh, boswellia, feverfew, turmeric, devil's claw, ginger, yucca, barberry, flaxseed oil, and fresh greens. Commercial formulas of these and other herbs can be tried for up to two to three weeks, or as suggested on labels. Popular herbal formulas often contain boswellia or turmeric as their principal herbs. Zyflamend is a superb herbal combination made by New Chapter. This formula, currently under major scientific study, can help arthritis and other inflammations.

Rheumatoid arthritis, a painful and potentially debilitating kind of arthritis, is related to underlying inflammation (see line of defense 4). Seriously consider supplementation with omega-3 fatty acids. Anyone with this condition needs professional advice about diet, nutrition, and supplements.

Also consult Osteoarthritis and the Bones, later in this chapter.

Asthma: The primary symptoms of asthma are tightness in the chest, shortness of breath, and wheezing. The bronchioles in the lungs, which are like little pipes, become narrower. There are several causes of asthma, including allergies and environmental pollutants. Asthma is most definitely a disease that involves inflammation and stress. Consult lines of defense 2 and 4. Asthma can also indicate underlying weakness in the body. Consult line of defense 1. If you are on asthma medication, do not reduce or get off medication without the advice of a physician. Asthma, and the shortness of breath, is a condition that needs care and expert guidance.

Asthma is on the rise in this country, tragically in children. With the multiple emotional stresses and proinflammatory diet, this is no surprise. Pharmaceutical drug use for this condition has ballooned in the past decades. Omega-3 fatty acid deficiency is certainly one factor in this rising problem, as well as the tendency to consume the white-food diet. Excess dairy, white flour three meals daily, few fresh vegetables, and saturated fats—a recipe for inflammation, allergies, and asthma.

Herbalists use a variety of herbal medicines for asthma, including elecampane, licorice, mullein, and red clover. Acupuncture can relieve stress and improve breathing.

In this chapter consult Allergies, Cleansing, Sinusitis, Cough, and Stress.

Atherosclerosis: A narrowing and hardening of the arteries, a common condition, is related to faulty diet, inflammation, and stress. Please consult lines of defense 1, 2, 3, and 4. Excess saturated fats, hydrogenated fats, and free radicals have a major role in hardening and thickening of the blood vessels. We want to keep our blood vessels clear and clean. In this chapter, see Heart and Cardiovascular.

Some major herbs for the blood vessels include hawthorn berry, ginkgo, garlic, artichoke, and red sage. See a health professional. Vitamin E and coenzyme Q_{10} may be suggested. Often, 100 mg of coenzyme Q_{10} daily is recommended.

Attention Deficit Disorder (ADD): A complex modern problem requiring the advice of a medical practitioner trained in nutritional and holistic medicine. Diet and nutrition play major roles in treating this condition, as well as strategies to relieve stress. See lines of defense 1, 2, and 3. Detoxification has a major role in potential treatment for this condition. Omega-3 deficiency, common in American teenagers, might be a major factor underlying this troubling problem.

The incredible proliferation of chemicals in medicines, food, and water, as well as household cleaning products, has some relation to the epidemic of this and related health problems. For treatment, seek the appropriate health professional.

Acupuncture, various stress-reduction techniques, and tender care are helpful adjunct strategies.

Back Pain: Short term. Many Americans suffer from back pain. Most short-term back pain is due to muscular tension. See advice under line of defense 2 and Sciatica in this chapter. A small percentage of back pain is due to a disk problem or a physical disability that might require a thorough medical examination.

Common causes of short-term back pain are:

* Poor posture
* Nervous tension and anger
* Falling or lifting a heavy object inappropriately
* Sitting too much (aggravated by poor posture)
* Not enough stretching

For those who are prone to muscle spasms and back pain, stretching is an important tool (see appendix 4). Stretching, however, is not as easy as it sounds. There are specific stretches that relieve tension in specific muscles. One should not stretch if in severe pain or if the stretching causes pain. The idea is to relax the muscle constriction around the area of pain. Often, professional advice about stretching is a necessity. Physical

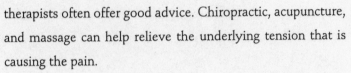

therapists often offer good advice. Chiropractic, acupuncture, and massage can help relieve the underlying tension that is causing the pain.

Recurring back pain is often due to negative attitudes and feedback. *"It's going to happen again. Every time I am pissed off, my back goes out."* The repetition of negative states and attitudes can precede the back's "going out."

Bacterial Infections: Harmful bacteria can afflict any part or organ of the body and often produce symptoms with fever, inflammation, redness, swelling, and pain. Any suspected bacterial infections need to be examined by a doctor. Specific foods and herbal medicines can support the immune system and decrease inflammation and pain, but these should not be used as a substitute for antibiotics unless prescribed by a physician. For stronger resistance, consult line of defense 5. And for better overall health, which supports immune response, see lines of defense 1, 2, and 3. When the immune system is strong, harmful bacteria are less likely to flourish. I have known people who rarely get bacterial infections.

Common herbal medicines that inhibit infections include echinacea, goldenseal, garlic, andrographis, turmeric, licorice, olive leaf, uva ursi, and oregano. See appendix 3. Also consult Cleansing in this chapter. An excellent herbal formula is the combination of echinacea and goldenseal: liquid extracts, 20 to 40 drops three times daily (short-term use only).

When taking antibiotics, take extra vitamin C and probiotics. See appendix 2 for information related to probiotics.

Bladder: See Urinary Tract Infections.

Blood Pressure: Hypertension. Sometimes called a silent killer, hypertension often has few detectible symptoms until complications start to develop. Extra pressure in the blood vessels puts pressure on the overworked heart, which has to pump blood to all the tissues of the body.

High blood pressure that goes on for too long taxes the heart and kidneys and can lead to diseases of those organs. Strokes can also occur—a bursting of a blood vessel in the brain, resulting in paralysis of a part of the body or even death. Blood pressure needs to be checked periodically, particularly for those who are smokers, overweight, and prone to high stress.

Advanced hypertension will produce an array of intense symptoms: headaches, rapid pulse, sweating, shortness of breath, and dizziness. Primary hypertension is not due to any underlying disease; its causes are numerous: smoking, excess stress, obesity, excessive use of stimulants like coffee, excessive use of salt. Nervous stress and tension cause the walls of the blood vessels to constrict. See line of defense 2. Internal and low-grade inflammation is also a factor to seriously consider (see line of defense 4).

Secondary hypertension is due to specific underlying physical causes, the most common being Atherosclerosis (see that heading in this chapter).

High blood pressure needs the guidance of a qualified health practitioner. However, stress, toxification, and inflammation can have a major role in causing this potentially dangerous condition.

Blood Vessels: See Atherosclerosis, and Heart and Cardiovascular.

Brain Health: See Memory.

Breasts: For female health and the health of the breast, there are many natural strategies. See lines of defense 1, 2, and 3. Stretching, yoga, and other body tune-up techniques are highly recommended. In Oriental medicine, detoxification of the liver is considered key in maintaining good breast health. Consult herbs under Female Remedies and Menstruation. Diet, stress reduction, and exercise are important considerations. Major herbs include dandelion root, motherwort, bupleurum, vitex (chaste berry), dong quai (also spelled dang gui), and flaxseed oil. A cleansing strategy for the breast might also include alternating red clover with dandelion root. Herbs that cleanse the liver are often one strategy that an herbalist will consider because in Oriental medicine the liver acupuncture meridian runs right through the breasts. Supplements include green supplements, green foods, evening primrose oil, vitamin E, alpha lipoic acid, and coenzyme Q_{10}.

Bronchitis: See Cough.

Bursitis: A painful joint problem due to inflammation of the bursa, the fluid-filled sac within the joint. See Tendinitis. Bursitis can be caused by occupational hazards such as working on your knees on a hard surface, resulting in bursitis in the knees. Housemaid's knee was a quaint old-fashioned diagnosis for bursitis that affects the knees. The prevention here is to protect the knees with pads and to shift positions while working. Also, consult lines of defense 1, 2, and 3.

Cancer: There are many different kinds of cancer, and two major divisions: benign or malignant. Malignant cancer, of prime interest in this section, is dangerous because it can spread and lead to death. Dr. Slaga said, in his book *The Detox Revolution,* "Cancer results from the complex interaction of many factors related to our environment, lifestyle, diet and genetic makeup." Since many cancers are directly related to faulty diet and certain foods, see the lines of defense 1 and 3. The foods to avoid: those that cause toxification and inflammation, particularly poor-quality fats, excess chemicals, and excess sugar. Carefully study line of defense 4. It is extremely important to keep the liver healthy. It is equally important to keep the intestines healthy and to support a strong immune system (see line of defense 5). Anyone with cancer should see a health professional if he or she wants to benefit from natural medicine.

Herbal medicines can be very helpful in preventing cancer and for treatment as an adjunct—with professional guidance. Some herbal medicines that might prevent cancer include maitake, reishi, burdock, dark leafy greens, red clover, pau d'arco, barberry, gynostemma, andrographis, schisandra, and omega-3 fatty acids in flaxseed and borage seed.

In *The Detox Revolution*, Dr. Slaga says, "Cancer development is usually a very slow process that often takes place over a period of years or even decades. The length of time (latency) to cancer formation depends on a number of factors such as genetics; the length of time of carcinogenic exposure; detoxification capabilities; DNA repair capacity; immune system strength; as well as diet, lifestyle, and age."

In Oriental medicine, cancer is related to faulty diet, organ imbalances (particularly the liver), and a variety of emotional stresses. Prolonged negative emotions can have a role to play in the genesis of cancer, creating inflammation and stagnation, which in time can become a tumor. Particularly harmful are chronic fear and anger. See line of defense 2. Meditative prayer, relaxation techniques, forgiveness, acceptance, and creative visualization techniques can be a part of a positive healing path. Therapies that support overall energy and well-being include acupuncture, network chiropractic, polarity therapy, reiki, and chi kung. Chi kung is an Oriental healing exercise that nourishes and supports the whole body and is highly recommended for cancer patients.

Carpal Tunnel Syndrome: This is now a common source of pain due to repetitive strain, often from working on computers. Most commonly the median nerve in the wrist becomes compressed, causing local pain in wrist and hands, numbness, and sometimes tingling. This is a local inflammation due to injury. After a medical exam there are several good solutions. Watch your posture when you work the hand. Gentle stretching of the hand, wrist, and arm can be very helpful, as long as the pain is not aggravated. Professional advice can be especially helpful. While working at a computer, get up occasionally and stretch, squeeze a tennis ball, and relax the neck and shoulders. Tight neck and shoulders are almost always involved in the genesis of this pain. A good solution in the early

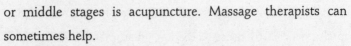

or middle stages is acupuncture. Massage therapists can sometimes help.

Vitamin B-complex can be helpful as well as the herbs yucca, boswellia, and bromelain, which reduce swelling and pain.

Self-massage is very helpful. Don't hurt yourself! Gently massage the forearm and wrist area with arnica ointment every day. Massage the pericardium 6 point, two inches up from the wrist crease on the palm side of the forearm.

Chemical Toxicity: Anyone who has been exposed to toxic chemicals should see a physician. Consult line of defense 3. Two safe detoxifying herbal medicines are milk thistle and schisandra.

Chronic Fatigue: In this stressed-out world with a plethora of debilitating foods and drugs, there are many opportunities for energy crashing. Many people with chronic fatigue are suffering from long-term energy burnout. They usually have lit the candle at both ends for several years. Consult line of defense 1. Many people suffer from prolonged stress and overwork (see line of defense 2). Consult with a health professional about adding to your improved nutrition one of the following herbal medicines: ginseng, ashwagandha, rhodiola, or gynostemma. Some herbalists call this condition adrenal exhaustion.

Consult Fatigue and Exhaustion in this chapter. Some other solutions include herbal medicine, acupuncture, yoga, stress-reduction techniques like biofeedback and meditation, yoga, tai chi, and chi kung.

I have treated this condition over the past twenty years and have offered patients a comprehensive strategy: nutritional guidance, herbal medicines, and acupuncture. However, the essential strategy is for the patient to engage in a sensible and consistent path of self-healing, which includes eating well, pacing oneself (and not overdoing it), and engaging in several proactive health strategies, which are mentioned above.

Cleansing: In traditional holistic medicine, cleansing is another term for detoxification. See line of defense 3. While all traditional systems of medicine, including Oriental, include different kinds of cleansing as a fundamental part of their medical practice, current Western medicine has no such strategy—a great loss. The facts provided in the five lines of defense amply testify to the importance of proper elimination, healthy detoxification by the liver, and reduction of inflammation. Many diseases have their root in "toxic conditions" of the body, and much pain and disease can be prevented by following the simple rules of detoxification as outlined in line of defense 3.

Signs of toxification do not necessarily manifest in disease, though in time diseases can result. Prior to the signs of disease, the following symptoms can predominate: sluggishness, malaise, fatigue, headaches, irregular or few bowel movements, irritability, digestive problems, swollen glands, bloating, gas, and poor sleep.

There are many foods and herbs that assist in detoxification. Some of the major ones include pau d'arco, schisandra, gynostemma, turmeric, goldenseal, dandelion, bupleurum, barberry, green tea, echinacea, andrographis, and red clover. Herbalists often use synergistic herbal formulas depending on the symptoms presented by the patient. A synergistic herbal formula is a mixture of herbs that work well together and have been used for decades. Two of the most famous cleansing formulas in America today are the essiac and Hoxsey formulations. In Ayurvedic medicine, there are several major formulas, including triphala. A common Oriental formula for gentle detoxification is the bupleurum and dong quai (dang gui; free and easy wanderer), available in capsules or tablets at better health food stores.

Common Cold: The common cold is more liable to manifest when you are tired and run down. For prevention of colds, see advice under line of defense 1. Several vitamins and herbs either prevent colds or enhance the healing of colds: vitamin C with bioflavonoids, zinc, echinacea, ginger extract or strong tea, and ginseng. For recurrent colds, consult the advice under line of defense 5.

If considering an herb like echinacea, take it three times daily for a few days as soon as symptoms commence. Colds, especially the damp and chilly ones with fluent clear discharge, respond well to frequent warm herbal teas—ginger tea is a good one. Garlic, echinacea, and ginger are cold preventatives. A common European tea is a combination of elder flower, peppermint, and yarrow. Another favorite is the liquid extract of echinacea and goldenseal—short-term use only. Place 15 to 20 drops in juice or water three times a day, preferably right at the start of a cold—or even before! Remember, some herbs are contraindicated for long-term use (see appendix 3). Recurrent colds can respond to astragalus formulas.

Constipation: Consult lines of defense 1, 2, and 3. While the primary cause of constipation lies in diet, stress and tension can aggravate this condition. For the most part, bowel movements should occur every day. Constipation can result in toxification and poor energy, as well as susceptibility to diseases. Toxification is hard on the liver, quality of blood, and general health. It is therefore imperative to have regular bowel movements. Movement through the intestines is created by a wave of movement in the walls, peristalsis. This movement is helped by a variety of fiber foods, which have bulk and roughage. It is best to eat a variety of fiber foods: different kinds of vegetables, fruits, grains, and beans.

Recommended are:

1. A diet with plenty of fiber—fruits, whole grains, vegetables, and water. Please remember that people who have consumed a refined-flour diet with little fiber must move into a high-fiber diet slowly.

2. Herbs, including senna and buckthorn, which contain chemicals that really do stimulate the bowels. Use these cautiously or as directed by a health professional. Psyllium is a seed that expands when moist and increases bowel motility.

3. Prunes, which are a gentle laxative.

4. Exercise, especially vigorous movement, is important.

5. Consulting a drug reference book, doctor, or pharmacist regarding medical drugs, antihistamines, diuretics, and antidepressants as some can cause constipation.

6. Avoiding excess white-flour products, refined foods, and junk foods, which can all contribute to lazy bowels.

7. Avoiding habitual use of laxatives, which can complicate constipation, creating chronic bowel problems.

8. Slowing down. People always in a rush, who leave little time for body care, are particularly susceptible to constipation.

Probiotics are often a good supplement for chronic bowel problems, especially for those who have taken certain pain-reducing drugs and antibiotics. See line of defense 2. Triphala is a good herbal formula for cleansing and longevity. Stretching can be helpful, particularly stretches for the lower abdomen. Often people hold tension and fear there. See appendix 4 on stretching. Five minutes of deep breathing can help.

Caution: Any person with chronic bowel problems should consult a physician before taking any herbal medicines or starting a high-fiber diet. Any chronic constipation or changes of color in bowels or bleeding can be a warning to see a physician.

Cough: Coughing is one of the major symptoms of distressed lungs. The respiratory system is highly susceptible to poor-quality air, chemicals, and pollutants and can be greatly assisted by good nutrition. Consult line of defense 1.

Most coughing is a common reflex action of the body, often the result of cold, flu, or allergy, but some persistent or violent coughs are warning signs that should be heeded. Consult a physician. Herbal teas and syrups can soothe simple coughs and support the lungs and immune system. Common herbs that support the respiratory system include English ivy, red clover, elderberry, oregano, elecampane, gynostemma, usnea, licorice, thyme, schisandra, hyssop, yarrow, and yerba santa. English ivy is used for repetitive spasmodic cough. Dr. Rudolph Weiss, a prominent German physician, gives the following herbal tea for acute dry coughs: equal parts mullein, coltsfoot, marshmallow, and anise seed to make 2 teaspoons in a cup of boiling water. Cover and infuse for twenty minutes and drink several times a day, with honey if desired. For dry, weak persistent coughs: American ginseng. For thick mucus coughs: elecampane or elderberry formulas. Other good formulas contain oregano, hyssop, thyme, cherry bark, or mullein.

See your doctor if the cough lasts for more than seven days, or if there is rusty, green, or yellow phlegm; high fever; shortness of breath; body aches; weight loss; chest pains; or severe headache. Coughing blood requires a medical exam.

To expand the lungs and relax the chest cavity, try daily stretching: just ten to fifteen minutes. See appendix 4.

Crohn's Disease: This condition requires the expert advice of a qualified holistic health professional if one is seeking alternatives from conventional medicine. Like colitis, Crohn's disease is related to long-term inflammation in the bowels (consult Ulcerative Colitis, which is quite similar to Crohn's disease). Remember that certain drugs and foods can instigate inflammation in the bowels, as well as chronic constipation. Probiotics are often needed for bowel health because of insult by faulty diet or medications. Please consult Constipation, as well as lines of defense 1 and 3.

Depression: Moderate depression can be helped by advice in lines of defense 1 and 2. In Oriental medicine it is said that to be happy one must have enough energy. Vitality and stamina are fundamental in preventing unnecessary depression. However, keep in mind that almost everyone has days when they are down and blue.

Some causes of mild or moderate depression include:

* Sugar blues. Try improving the diet and greatly reducing sugar.
* Emotional and family problems.
* Diet: see line of defense 1.
* A variety of life stresses all hitting at once: see line of defense 2.
* Not enough friendship. Get out and meet people, join groups and social activities.

See a physician for deep chronic depression, marked by daily apathy, lethargy, and lack of focus.

Supplements to consider with a health professional are Saint-John's-wort, which is the principal choice, but also ginseng, ashwagandha, omega-3 fatty acids, and specific vita-

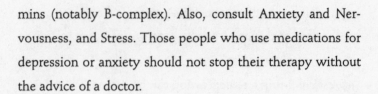

mins (notably B-complex). Also, consult Anxiety and Nervousness, and Stress. Those people who use medications for depression or anxiety should not stop their therapy without the advice of a doctor.

Diabetes (Adult Onset): A disease of inflammation and stress, caused partially by faulty diet, particularly refined carbohydrates and sugar. Please consult lines of defense 1, 2, and 4. Most people who become diabetic in adulthood are overweight, which contributes to inflammation in the body. Diabetes is a problem that is very common in countries where people eat too much rich food, sugar, and other products of a prosperous civilization. See Diseases of Civilization. Consult with your physician if you are on medication and make any changes to your dietary regime. Cinnamon, and other herbs, can be used to lower blood-sugar levels, but this is best done with professional guidance.

Diarrhea: Emotional distress and reactions to food and medications are the primary causes of short-term diarrhea. Diarrhea can be one way that the body decides to eliminate toxins and inflammation. If the body needs to detoxify and eliminate excess heat, it is best not to mess with it. Kaopectate is a common remedy that can be purchased at the pharmacy. Herbs that can ease simple cases include psyllium, red raspberry, bilberry, ginger, or chamomile. Slippery elm is a soothing herb for the intestines. Recommended foods include raw green apples, bananas, papaya, applesauce, oats, and yogurt. Milk products can be allergenic, as can wheat products. Ingest yogurt or acidophilus for diarrhea brought on by antibiotics or reactions to food. Cautions: Diarrhea that lasts for more than a few days, as well as bloody, painful, or violent diarrhea, prompts the need for a medical exam. Recurrent diarrhea can be a sign of irritable bowel syndrome (alternating with constipation), colitis, or gastroenteritis (diarrhea alternating with vomiting). See a physician.

Diseases of Civilization: In modern countries like America, many of our primary diseases are results of living in a comfortable and affluent civilization. We often eat too much and eat the wrong kinds of foods: comfort foods, which are generally sugary, fatty, and white—sometimes salty. This poor-quality diet of excess, combined with lack of exercise, contributes to arthritis, cancer, heart problems, immune weakness, and a host of other diseases. Key areas stressed in the body include the intestines, liver, and immune system, and often a low-key, hard-to-detect systemic inflammation occurs, resulting in such problems as joint pain, high cholesterol, and headaches. See all five lines of defense. In this chapter consult Cleansing, Constipation, Stress, and Fatigue and Exhaustion.

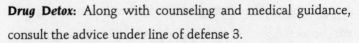

Drug Detox: Along with counseling and medical guidance, consult the advice under line of defense 3.

Herbalists will use some of the following herbs: ashwagandha, Saint-John's-wort, milk thistle, and schisandra. These herbs have different functions, so consult an herbal specialist.

Dyspepsia: See Indigestion.

Eczema: See Skin.

Environmental Sensitivity: Some people are overly sensitive to chemicals, molds, and odors. This is a condition for a professional but is almost always related to toxification (particularly the bowels), stress, and a compromised immune system. Also consult lines of defense 1 through 5.

A condition known as leaky bowel syndrome is sometimes related to this troubling disorder. The walls of the intestine become so inflamed and stressed that toxins leak back into the body, causing an array of symptoms. Consult Leaky Bowel Syndrome in this chapter.

Eyes: This refers to eye strain, itchy eyes, and general health. The eyes are susceptible to air pollutants, dust, and wind. Lutein, a phytochemical in certain plants, improves vision.

Foods rich in certain phytochemicals can help eye health, such as most berries. For long-term eye health see lines of defense 1, 2, and 3. In Oriental medicine, the health of the eyes is related to the liver (consult Cleansing). Some herbs to consider are dandelion root, milk thistle, and bilberry. Supplements that are recommended for eye health include coenzyme Q_{10}, vitamin A, omega-3 fatty acids, and green foods like spirulina.

Fatigue and Exhaustion: Consult lines of defense 1 and 2. Much fatigue evolves from just plain overdoing it. Common terms include burnout or adrenal exhaustion. This section relates to fatigue or exhaustion related to athletes who overdo it or anyone burdened by a period of too much work or distress. Common sense about a healthy diet and not too many stimulants is important: Too much coffee, rich food/sugar, and lack of sleep can lead to fatigue. Of course, excess emotional and mental stress can be a major factor.

A doctor should examine a case of fatigue that is long-term or recurrent. Chronic fatigue or exhaustion unrelated to overwork, restless sleep, or excess exercise could be a warning sign sending us to a physician. Long-term emotional distress can also result in fatigue, a situation that might require counseling or medical care. In herbal medicine, long-term tiredness can be related to poor organ functioning, such as an overburdened liver or intestine. An herbalist might diagnose a congested liver and prescribe two to three weeks of special diet and liver cleansing herbs.

Herbal medicines to consider include the ginsengs, gotu kola, and astragalus. Saint-John's-wort is helpful, particularly for those who are moderately depressed; it is often recommended in standardized tablets, 300 mg three times daily. For more advice about the assistance of our plant allies, see an appropriate health professional. Also see appendix 3.

Deep relaxation can be a great assistance in charging the batteries, as well as moderate exercise and stretching. See line of defense 2, as well as appendix 4.

Female Remedies: Good diet and stress reduction can help women in many ways: beauty, energy, healthy skin, hormone cycles, sexual health, and well-being. Consult lines of defense 1 through 3.

Also consult Breasts, Menstruation, PMS, and Sex Drive. A common tonic in Oriental medicine, particularly for blood tonification, is dong quai (dang gui), and white peony, which also helps to lessen menstrual cramping. This common formula is available in capsules and tablets. Other common herbal remedies for general health include dong quai, vitex, black cohosh, white peony, camp bark, omega-3 fatty acids, and motherwort. Fish oil capsules, soft gels, can be taken two to three times daily (usually 2 to 3 capsules).

Fertility: This is a complex problem that can find support in natural medicine. Some infertility is related to long-standing inflammation and toxification. It can also be related to insufficient energy. See a health professional trained in nutrition and herbal medicine and consult lines of defense 1, 2, 3, and 4.

Some people have been helped by acupuncture and herbal medicines. Herbal medicines to consider include those herbs listed under male or female issues (consult with your herbalist). Among the herbs that herbalists value are ginseng, gynostemma, saw palmetto, epimedium, and dong quai.

Fever: The suggestions provided here are for short-term low fevers, many of which are part of a healing response by the body. Fever can be a way of ridding the body of excess inflammation and toxins. Drink plenty of fluids, including herbal teas: echinacea, elderflower, peppermint, or chamomile. If a tea is made from one or a combination of these herbs, make it strong and drink a modest amount several times through the course of the day. Rest and reduce greasy and spicy foods. Most often it is best to let a moderate fever run its course without too much tampering with drugs, but fevers, especially with children, must be watched carefully. A cool compress on the forehead as well as a tepid upper-body wash can help cool the body. Make sure you keep a thermometer in your medicine cabinet because fevers over 102 degrees need monitoring and possible medical attention.

Fibromyalgia: A stubborn and challenging condition involving long-term wandering muscle pains, it is often hard to diagnose, unpredictable, and changeable, baffling doctors and patients. Often the patients are worse in the morning—stiff, achy, and suffering from pains here and there. There can be multiple causes: Going through a long period of stress and burnout is, in my experience, a common denominator in this problem. Faulty diet, constipation, and emotional distress are other common causative factors. Bowel problems can be a factor (see Cleansing, Constipation, Fatigue and Exhaustion, and Leaky Gut Syndrome).

Oriental medicine states that a subtle heat trapped in the muscle layers, manifesting in specific acupuncture points, causes this problem, most notably on the neck, shoulders, midback, and thighs. This subtle, low-grade inflammation is a sign that the body's overall energy is deficient—just not a lot of energy in the machine. One could say that fibromyalgia involves a low-key inflammation due to diet and stress. Consult lines of defense 1 through 3. For a solid program to turn this condition around, see the appropriate health professional.

Some advice that I tell my patients: Avoid excess sugar and too much caffeine, get adequate sleep, and exercise moderately three to five times weekly. In many patients with fibromyalgia, absorption of energy from food has been compromised (see advice under Fatigue and Exhaustion; many patients with fibromyalgia have gone through a long period of burning the candle at both ends). Many herbalists use adaptogenic herbs like ginseng, gynostemma, or ashwagandha alone or in formulas, but often a complete constitutional workup produces several therapeutic strategies. While there are no easy answers, a good holistic strategy can help patients completely recover from this stubborn and debilitating condition. A typical dose of Siberian gingseng would be 1 to 2 capsules or tablets two to three times daily.

Flu: Symptoms of flu are inflammation, a sign that the immune system is trying to fight off the invader. One is more susceptible to flu when one is run down and tired (see lines of defense 1 and 2). Often susceptibility to flu is enhanced by a subtle toxic condition in the body (see line of defense 3). Certainly fear and panic around the flu do not help people. For better confidence and resistance, please consult line of defense 5.

A virus, of which there are two major strains, causes A and B flu, also called influenza. The A flu is a more intense variant of the common cold. The symptoms are too well known: fever, chills, muscle aches, headache, weakness, and nasal discharge. The body can produce immunity to the flu virus. A common threat, as in the recent SARS, is the mutation of a virus in domestic animals and its release into the unsuspecting human population. The flu virus can be spread through coughing and sneezing and is particularly harmful in closed environments like office buildings and airplanes. While vaccines can be helpful to reduce the occurrence of influenza, they will not help in the recurring occurrence of mutated viruses. Some people respond poorly to these vaccines. Modern drugs can offer some relief, mostly from discomfort and pain.

Herbal medicines can help recovery from a flu faster, and if taken in time can prevent a flu from occurring. My favorite flu remedy is a blend of echinacea and elderberry, taken three times daily for a few days at the onset of symptoms. Other solutions include adding vitamin C with bioflavonoids and zinc two to three times daily. When using the herbs, the sooner the better, but they can also be taken a few days ahead of time if flu is in the neighborhood. Olive leaf extract is said to stimulate the immune system and inhibit viral infection.

Gas: Flatulence can be corrected by eating slower and consuming a sensible, balanced diet. Eating while emotionally upset will help instigate digestive wind! Eating on the run is definitely not recommended, nor is indugling in fiber-rich foods. See lines of defense 1 and 2.

Herbs that calm stomach and intestines include fennel, coriander, and caraway—all common kitchen herbs. Chamomile and peppermint, two common herbs, are good for many problems of the digestive system. Charcoal tablets, available at health food stores, are a universal standby. One can also ingest a small amount of burnt toast. Acidophilus can be used, particularly for those who have taken antibiotics. Food allergies, laxatives, antacids, antibiotics, and other drugs can disrupt the digestive system. Chronic gas accompanied by any pains, weight loss, fever, and swelling needs medical attention.

Recurrent bloating and gas, with irregular bowel movements and malaise, can be due to several problems relating to the ecology of the intestines, sometimes resulting from medications (particularly overuse of antibiotics), too many pain pills, and faulty diet. For more information, please consult Constipation and Leaky Gut Syndrome.

Gum Disease: Gum disease is a classic sign of inflammation: swollen, tender, and bleeding gums. Please consult lines of defense 1 through 4. Faulty nutrition (proinflammatory foods, in particular), poor dental hygiene, and excess nervous stress are often factors in the genesis of this stubborn problem.

Some helpful natural remedies include coenzyme Q_{10}, red clover formulas (to nourish the gums), bloodroot formulas (to rinse the mouth out), and goldenseal mouthwash, which is very cleansing. Also helpful are vitamin C with B-complex vitamins, calcium, and magnesium.

Hay Fever: See Allergies.

Headaches: For simple everyday stress headaches, the following remedies can offer positive relief. Also, consult line of defense 2. With many tension headaches, the scalp and neck become tight and tense. To relieve this tension, peruse these suggestions:

❋ Acupressure on the neck, shoulders, and scalp. Apply gentle circular pressure with fingertips, best done by a massage therapist or acupuncturist.

❋ Gentle stretching. See *Stretching* by Bob Anderson. Never overstretch the neck. Also consult appendix 4.

❋ Warm, relaxing lavender or rosemary baths.

❋ Feverfew or strong chamomile tea.

❋ A few drops of peppermint oil rubbed in the area of pain—avoid the eyes.

Any stubborn, long-term, or painful headaches require a medical examination.

Also see Migraine Headaches and Stress.

Heart and Cardiovascular: Good nutrition and stress reduction can have a beneficial effect on the heart and blood vessels. Many problems with the heart begin with long-term inflammation. Consult lines of defense 1 through 4. Anyone with suspected or diagnosed heart or blood pressure problems should consult a physician before using methods suggested in this book.

One of the favorite herbs for the heart is hawthorn berry. Coenzyme Q_{10} is also helpful. Stay away from hydrogenated oils, trans fats, and excess saturated fats. Consume foods like fish and green leafy vegetables. In this chapter consult Angina, Atherosclerosis, and Cleansing.

Heartburn: A common inflammation, most often set off by rushing when eating, eating acidic foods, and eating when stressed. Please consult lines of defense 1 through 4. Fried foods, too much spicy food, and excess citrus and tomato products are common culprits. Symptoms include a burning sensation in the stomach or throat, belching, and bloating. Quite clearly this is another health problem with an inflammatory background.

Helpful are digestive enzymes, sensible eating habits, and not eating on the run or when emotionally upset. One favorite soothing supplement is papaya tablets, or the fruit, as well as licorice herb (restricted for those with high blood pressure) and chamomile tea. Often people take too many antacids, which often contain toxic metals. Also consult Indigestion.

Hemorrhoids: This uncomfortable health problem is too common in American adults. Bulging veins around the anus and rectum cause pain and discomfort. This condition is often caused by a sedentary lifestyle, obesity, and faulty diet. Constipation and straining while having bowel movements are also main causative factors.

See Cleansing and Constipation. Also consult lines of defense 1, 2, and 3. Detoxification is often necessary if you want to cure this problem. Learn about good-quality fiber foods and eat a wide variety: root vegetables, apples, peas, whole-wheat bread, dried fruit, brown rice, oatmeal, prunes, green leafy vegetables, and beans. Avoid as much as possible white-flour products and anything that makes the bowels sluggish and constipated. The American fast-food and the white-food diet create many unnecessary and troublesome health problems.

Hepatitis: One of the prime symptoms of all strains of hepatitis is inflammation. See recommendations under lines of defense 3 and 4, but be cognizant of the fact that hepatitis needs medical attention.

Hepatitis is an inflammation of the liver. Excess alcohol, abuse of medical drugs, and exposure to poisonous chemicals can cause inflammation of the liver, but it is most commonly caused by a viral infection. There are several viruses that can cause hepatitis, the most dangerous being B and C. The most serious kinds are caused by infusions of tainted blood, sexual contact, and drug users sharing needles. Symptoms vary but most common are malaise, fatigue, flulike symptoms, and loss of appetite. Later jaundice, fever, nausea, headache, swollen joints, and other symptoms can evolve.

When the liver cannot detoxify the blood properly, a host of serious symptoms ensues. Herbal medicines can help all forms of hepatitis, but only with the advice of a professional. Herbal medicines can interact with drug therapy used for hepatitis so it is important not to self-medicate for this disease. A healthy diet—low in saturated fats, junk foods, and chemicals—can nourish the ailing liver, which responds well to fresh greens, lemons, and fruits, all rich in phytonutrients and vitamins. Herbal medicines that are commonly used are milk thistle, bupleurum (in Oriental herbal formulas), licorice, schisandra, and goldenseal.

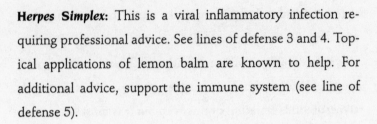

Herpes Simplex: This is a viral inflammatory infection requiring professional advice. See lines of defense 3 and 4. Topical applications of lemon balm are known to help. For additional advice, support the immune system (see line of defense 5).

High Cholesterol: High cholesterol can lead to problems and diseases of the blood vessels and heart. In Oriental medicine we consider high cholesterol a symptom of inflammation and toxification, often due to negative emotions, stress, liver abuse, and overwork. Inflammation derives from proinflammatory diet and high stress (examine lines of defense 1 through 4).

A physician should monitor people with high cholesterol. If the natural methods do not lower the cholesterol, medications are the best solution.

Cholesterol drugs often do not get to the root of the problem. Along with dietary changes, exercise, stress reduction, and medical checkups, an herbalist may prescribe the following herbs: garlic, guggul, psyllium, green tea, he shou wu, shiitake, or fenugreek. Some quality companies manufacture herbal/vitamin formulas for high cholesterol, available at good health food stores.

Acupuncture can help with the stress and detoxification. Massage can be a good addition to a therapeutic program.

Yoga, martial arts, tai chi, various kinds of exercise, and meditation can also be of great assistance. Also consult Cleansing, Diseases of Civilization, and Heart and Cardiovascular.

HIV/AIDS: See lines of defense 1 through 5 for adjunct care while under medical supervision. Certainly, HIV has many red flags that point to chronic and debilitating inflammation. Much helpful advice can be found in the five lines of defense, but to really benefit from a natural, holistic approach, turn to the appropriate health professional.

Immune System: Please consult line of defense 5. The immune system is a complex of factors that protect us from disease factors like pernicious bacteria, viruses, and parasites. Abuses to the immune system are very common in the modern world: recreational drugs, overuse of medical drugs, pollution, excess emotional distress, electromagnetic pollution, inadequate nutrition, and a diet rich in salt, saturated fats, and junk food. There are many strategies to strengthen the immune system. The most important are healthy nutrition, fresh air, exercise, and natural remedies. The immune system is intimately connected to the emotions and thoughts and can be greatly helped when our emotional/mental state is more harmonious and positive. Chronic worry, anger, overthinking, and anxiety can weaken the immune system, particularly when combined with an inadequate diet. When the intestines are not healthy, the immune system can be compromised. See Constipation, Leaky Gut Syndrome, and appendix 2 information about probiotics, supplements that are important for general health.

Herbal medicines that support the immune system include astragalus, elderberry, American ginseng, garlic, reishi, echinacea, schisandra, ligustrum, pau d'arco, red clover, and leafy greens. Astragalus formulas are highly recommended.

Nutritional supplements include spirulina, alpha lipoic acid, coenzyme Q_{10}, zinc, and vitamin E. Acidophilus is also important. Anyone with immune-related diseases should consult a professional before using herbal remedies.

Impotence: See lines of defense 1 through 3. This health problem can have a variety of causes, which might require the advice of a doctor, nutritionist, herbalist, or psychotherapist. For people who are wary of drug therapy, good results can result from a combination of acupuncture, improved nutrition, and herbal medicine (see Male Remedies and Sex Drive).

Indigestion: This is a generic term for quite a few very common stomach/intestinal ailments. This problem, like sinus and breathing problems, plagues busy urban Americans. Often food and air quality, as well as a hectic lifestyle, play havoc on the digestion. In fact, indigestion is one of the most common disorders that afflicts human beings. Symptoms can vary, but include gas, abdominal pains, heartburn, bloating, belching, vomiting, and mild nausea. Indigestion is most often diet related: eating too fast, while under emotional stress, or overindulging in rich food. Please consult lines of defense 1 through 3.

Some abdominal disorders are due to a little-known condition called Leaky Gut Syndrome, resulting in fatigue, occasional diarrhea, bloating, gas, poor digestion, and symptoms of general malaise. Consult Leaky Gut Syndrome in this chapter, particularly if you suffer from irritable bowel syndrome and related disorders, allergies, asthma, and inflamed joints.

Herbal remedies for the digestion are many. Chamomile is the standard, or peppermint (more for bloating and gas). Take it as a tea three times daily. A dependable all-around tea is peppermint/ginger. Swedish bitters, a traditional herbal formula, are used for poor stomach digestion and acid symptoms. Bitter herbal tonics have been used for hundreds of years to tone the digestive system.

Fennel, licorice, and fenugreek are other common herbal remedies for a stressed stomach. For chronic indigestion— after a medical checkup—seek stress relief through medita-

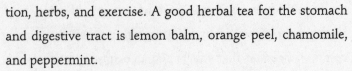

tion, herbs, and exercise. A good herbal tea for the stomach and digestive tract is lemon balm, orange peel, chamomile, and peppermint.

Caution: Any severe cramping, vomiting, pain, or digestive symptoms accompanied by fever, diarrhea, vomiting, bleeding, and any alterations of the color of stools could be a sign of a medical emergency.

Insect Bites and Stings: Here we have a classic sign of localized inflammation, caused by the body protecting itself. Some effective home remedies to apply externally include tea tree oil or garlic juice. Baking soda, moistened and applied to bites, is a good old home remedy. For a few very sensitive people, insect bites can be a medical emergency. Symptoms to watch out for are difficulty breathing, confusion, convulsions, loss of consciousness, rapid red swelling, or throat constriction.

Insomnia: See Sleeplessness.

Irritable Bowel Syndrome: This often requires the advice of a medical practitioner knowledgeable about foods and nutritional solutions. Improving eating patterns and reducing stress can help all bowel problems. Much helpful advice can be found in lines of defense 1 through 3. Irritable bowel syndrome is a symptom of inflammation and tension in the walls of the intestines, and the most common symptoms include bloating, gas, soreness, and alternation of diarrhea and constipation.

Some natural treatments to consider include enteric coated peppermint (1 to 2 capsules three times daily for the short term), flaxseeds, and strong chamomile tea. Emotional vexation is sometimes the cause of this problem, as well as poor dietary habits such as eating too fast, eating on the run, and eating when emotionally charged. Other natural strategies include Saint-John's-wort for relaxation, American ginseng, and 5-HTP (a natural supplement). Oriental herbalists will prescribe liver and digestive herbal formulas. Consult information about probiotics in appendix 2, because these supplements are essential for many bowel problems.

In this chapter, see Indigestion, Cleansing, Stress, Constipation, and Leaky Gut Syndrome.

Joints: See Arthritis and Sports Injuries/Muscle Strain.

Kidney: The kidneys filter and clean the liquids of the body. Like the liver, they help clean the body of toxins and wastes. The health of the kidneys is enhanced by adequate water, reduction of poor-quality fats, avoidance of excess chemicals, and the health of the liver, which cleans the blood. In this chapter, see Cleansing and examine lines of defense 1 through 3. Because the kidneys are closely related to the bladder, prob-

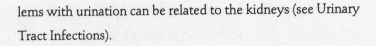

lems with urination can be related to the kidneys (see Urinary Tract Infections).

Leaky Gut Syndrome: This syndrome is not a disease. It is a low-grade inflammation and irritation that damages the walls of the small intestine. Leaky gut syndrome, not fully recognized yet, is far more common today than it should be and is often a factor in many chronic inflammations: fibromyalgia, environmental sensitivity, allergies, sinusitis, and irritable bowel syndrome. Faulty diet is one cause, particularly an excess of saturated and trans fats, white-flour products, and lack of vegetables. Consult line of defense 1. An aggravation of this problem is emotional and mental stress (consult line of defense 2). Perhaps the main cause is drugs, particularly NSAIDs and steroids. Another potential cause is chronic constipation (see that heading in this chapter).

The walls of the gut become more permeable, leaking toxins and wastes back into the body, not out of the body. The blood is infiltrated with a mass of impurities, creating systemic problems and inflammations. This messy situation can aggravate breathing, sinuses, lungs, liver, and the immune system, leading to long-term allergies, chemical and food sensitivities, gas and bloating, indigestion, fatigue, malaise, muscle aches, joint pain, confusion, brain fog, poor memory, skin rashes, mood changes, decreased immunity, and hyperactivity. See Constipation, Indigestion, and Irritable Bowel Syndrome in this chapter.

If you suspect that you suffer from this condition, please consult the book *Total Renewal* by Dr. Frank Lipman (see appendix 6) and seriously consider seeing an appropriate health professional.

Some helpful hints about healthful foods can be found in line of defense 1. Some useful supplements include licorice root, aloe vera juice, slippery elm herb, omega-3 fatty acids, and gamma-oryzanol.

Liver: See Cleansing and Drug Detox.

Longevity: Consult all five lines of defense in chapter 3. One can confidently say that good, wholesome nutrition, exercise, and a happy, creative heart and mind are the foundation of longevity. It has been found that most people who live long lives keep active and creative until their last days. Leafy greens, carrots, rice, beans, winter squash, green tea, soy products, turnips, and onions contain antioxidants that can slow the aging process. Recently it has been discovered that the folic acid in greens and beans can slow the onset of Alzheimer's disease. Excess saturated fats like margarine and some meat fats can harm the body in the long run. Fish oils, olive oil, primrose, and other good-quality oils are necessary nutritional supplements to ensure good health. For more complete dietary tips, carefully examine line of defense 1. Exercise that tones the joints, muscles, and heart is essential for a long life, as is continued flexibility of the spine through stretching, exercise, acupressure, and massage. The motility and health of the intestines, the quality of the blood, and the vigor of the immune system are of the utmost importance in promoting good health and long life. Processed foods, saturated fats, unnecessary chemical drugs, nicotine, excess caffeine, poor sex life, lack of sleep, overwork, negative emotions, and lack of exercise can undermine the health of the liver, blood, and body.

Some premier longevity herbs are ginseng, schisandra, reishi and maitake mushrooms, milk thistle, morinda, he shou wu, garlic, ginkgo, greens, rosemary, astragalus, eclipta, dong quai, epimedium, saw palmetto, green tea, and hawthorn. For more advice about herbal medicines and supplements, consult appendices 1, 2, and 3.

Supplements include acidophilus, coenzyme Q_{10}, alpha lipoic acid, glutathione, vitamin E, omega-3 fatty acids, zinc, and B-complex vitamins. The health of the bowels is essential for longevity (see Cleansing, Constipation, Irritable Bowel Syndrome, and Leaky Gut Syndrome).

Lungs: For improved health of the lungs, consult line of defense 1. Also, consult Immune System, Fatigue and Exhaustion, and Cleansing. The lungs breathe in the air, and the oxygen in the air is an essential fuel for the body. The pair of lungs is spongy and somewhat delicate and breathes in a host of pollutants from urban air. The lungs can also be an organ of elimination, particularly when we cough out mucus, dust, and other unwanted particles. The health of our lungs is helped by good nutrition rich in vitamins and antioxidants, as well as moderate exercise. Certain stretching exercises are helpful for opening up the lungs and allowing for deeper breathing. See appendix 4 on stretching.

Some supplements and foods that are particularly good for the lungs are ginger tea; ginger in cooking; vitamins A and C found in many fruits and vegetables; root vegetables like carrots, turnips, and burdock; coenzyme Q_{10}; garlic supplements; garlic; onions; cabbage; echinacea and goldenseal; elecampane herb; and green food supplements like spirulina. When the lungs are rundown and weak, we are more susceptible to colds, breathing problems, wheezing, phlegm, and bronchitis. For weak lungs, I suggest more rest, herbal teas, antioxidant vitamin supplements, and extra garlic. Another useful hint: Breathe in the healthful aroma of lung-clearing herbs such as peppermint, eucalyptus, and rosemary. Every home should

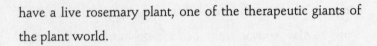

have a live rosemary plant, one of the therapeutic giants of the plant world.

Lyme Disease: This is a chronic inflammatory disease caused by bacteria that is transmitted by ticks. It is most common in the Northeast, where it is spread by deer that have infested open areas around the suburbs. Mice also carry the tick. Precautions must be taken when walking through fields, lawns, and forests. Wear the proper clothing and check carefully for ticks after an outdoor excursion. It is possible that people who contract Lyme had immune systems that could not eliminate the bacterial infection. For some helpful advice, consult lines of defense 1 through 5.

Lyme is a difficult disease to diagnose because its symptoms mimic other diseases. It often starts with a red "bullseye" rash at the site of the bite. If the bacteria penetrates the blood and is not killed by the immune system, fatigue, headache, muscle pain, and other symptoms can ensue. Untreated, the disease can develop into recurring arthritis. The prescribed antibiotic therapy, while necessary, can compromise the bowels and immune system.

Herbal medicine, best prescribed by a professional, can assist in the healing and offset the deleterious effect of the strong antibiotic therapy. Natural medicines to consider include astragalus formulas, baikal skullcap, mushrooms like shiitake extracts, licorice, pau d'arco, and red clover. These must be prescribed according to the specific needs of the patient. Also, for those who have antibiotic therapy, see the discussion of probiotics in appendix 2.

Male Remedies: There are many strategies to improve male health, and most of these can be found in all five lines of defense. For those who are seeking a boost of energy, more vigor, and stamina, herbal medicine is a safe and effective route. Some common herbs to consider with your health practitioner include saw palmetto, ginseng (all of them), ginkgo, milk thistle, garlic, he shou wu, rehmannia, damiana, muira puama, morinda, catuaba, and horny goat weed (epimidium). Sound nutrition, exercise, and herbal medicines are a safe, effective program for men seeking more energy and better health. Herbs like yohimbe, or medical drugs that arouse the sex drive, should be used cautiously because of possible long-term side effects. Herbal medicine can safely improve sex life, but quality of sexuality is dependent on essential factors such as affection, sensuality, and respect. Also, please refer to Sex Drive in this chapter.

Memory: In chapter 3 pay particular attention to line of defense 1, as well as lines of defense 3 and 4. Also, in this chapter consult Cleansing and Longevity.

To preserve good memory, a healthy diet rich in nutrients and antioxidants is necessary. Saturated fats, cigarette smoke, salt, and the "junky" foods are not good for the blood vessels that feed the brain. Omega-3 fatty acids are recommended for brain health. Herbs that are good for brain cell activity are quite a few. These include ginkgo, bacopa, gotu kola, ashwagandha, morinda, epimidium, hawthorn, garlic, and biota seed pill to nourish the heart (an Oriental formula). Supplements include green foods like spirulina, blue-green algae, alfalfa, as well as omega-3 fatty acids and alpha lipoic acid. Poor memory can be due to several energetic imbalances in the body: deficient nervous system, deficient energy, poor functioning liver, and stagnant or sluggish blood circulation. Prescribed foods and herbal formulas can address each or all of these problems. A typical recommendation would be 40 mg of ginkgo bilboa three times a day for three months.

Menopause: In some simple cultures, the symptoms of menopause are rare or nonexistent. Menopause can, along with other disharmonies (high blood pressure and cholesterol, for example), be considered a problem of a civilization. High levels of stress and faulty diet contribute to the genesis and intensity of this health problem. A good balanced diet, herbal medicines, and relaxation can really soften the intensity of symptoms. See lines of defense 1 and 2.

Nutrition is fundamental to correct the more unpleasant symptoms. Follow a diet high in vegetables, fish, fruits, soybean products, and high-fiber foods, and limit coffee and other stimulants, saturated fats, sugar, and junk foods.

Helpful remedies to consider: vitex, dong quai, vitamin E, motherwort, essential fatty acids, schisandra, red clover, black cohosh formulas, and unicorn root. Yoga, tai chi, acupuncture, and meditation are good adjunct tools. The natural passage of menopause can be greatly eased with good nutrition and herbal remedies. If you try an herb like black cohosh, which has quite a good reputation, use it for up to six weeks and if there is little improvement try another. My typical recommendation could include dong quai capsules three times daily and fish oil capsules (three daily) for three months.

Menstruation: Many menstrual problems are aggravated by stress, tension, and faulty diet. Please consult lines of defense 1 through 3 for some very helpful advice.

Many excellent foods and herbs exist for the health of women and the free passage of the menses. For prolonged painful and irregular menstrual cycles, it is good to consult a professional. Some herbs for a deficient menstrual cycle (amenorrhea) include dong quai, vitex, dandelion, nettle leaf extract, schisandra, myrrh, or red clover formulas. A vigorous and balanced diet is very important in a deficient menstrual cycle.

For pain and discomfort prior to or during menstrual cycles, producing cramping, lower backache, and, in severe cases, nausea and vomiting, common solutions include fatty acid supplementation; proper diet and nutrition with a limit on sugar, caffeine, saturated fats, alcohol, and meat products; and the regular inclusion of relaxation exercises, stretching, yoga, and chi kung. There are many natural remedies for your professional to consider: cramp bark formulas, dong quai (dang gui) formulas, white peony, motherwort, milk thistle, wild yam, vitex, and black cohosh root formulas. Oriental herbalists use red sage and dong quai formulas. Recommended, too, is a vitamin formula specifically for women containing minerals, B-complex vitamins, and antioxidants like vitamin E. In this chapter consult Female Remedies and PMS.

Migraine Headaches: A fairly common kind of intense headache that sometimes persists for several days, often accompanied by light sensitivity, nausea, and neck stiffness, they are more numerous in women than men. No one really knows what cause migraines, but the main source of the pain is changes in the diameter of the blood vessels of the scalp— they constrict and then dilate. Migraines are often related to changes in estrogen levels. These stubborn and debilitating headaches can be set off by a wide range of stress factors, such as arguments, changes in barometer, premenstrual changes, and certain foods. Please consult advice under line of defense 2.

Massage of the scalp and neck, particularly prior to the onset, is a good preventive measure, as is acupuncture and deep relaxation techniques. Foods that might set off a migraine include chocolate, aged cheeses, citrus fruits, sodium nitrates, MSG, and red wine.

Some nutrients and herbs that can help: magnesium, niacin, B-complex vitamins, and the herb feverfew. Feverfew can be taken in capsules or tablets two to three times daily for several weeks. Magnesium relaxes constricted blood vessels. In Germany, a pioneer in the use of herbal medicines, the herb petasites is used for migraines. Petasites should only be used if certified free of pyrrolizidine alkaloids. Some might consider visiting a homeopathist who will prescribe according to presenting symptoms and might consider remedies like belladonna or bryonia.

Certainly inflammation is an underlying factor in migraines, setting off inappropriate nerve responses that then affect the blood vessels. See lines of defense 1, 2, 3, and 4.

Mind: See Memory.

Multiple Sclerosis: This is a mysterious disease that damages the fatty sheath that covers the nerve fibers in the brain and spinal column, resulting in such symptoms as poor mobility, weak muscles, and slurred speech. Symptoms can fluctuate, and patients can go through months, even years, of remission. Although the cause of this disease is not known, many scientists now consider it an autoimmune disease. It is worth considering that the immune system is confused by underlying inflammation. A qualified holistic health professional can offer solutions that do not resort to strong drug therapy. Essential fatty acid supplementation is known to help some sufferers of this disease. Holistic health professionals offer a positive strategy involving supplements, exercise, and diet.

Muscle Spasm: See line of defense 2.

Muscle Weakness: By this I mean wilting or atrophying of the muscles. To give the body support, consult line of defense 1. Some cases of chronic muscle weakness could be related to toxins in the body (see line of defense 3). With any case of muscle weakness, always consult a physician. Chinese herbalists use formulas with herbs like ginseng, licorice, and rehmannia. See a professional. Acupuncture can be a good adjunct tool.

Neck Pain: Short-term neck stiffness and discomfort are very common problems. See the advice under Back Pain. Tensions in the neck and shoulders are closely connected and much helped by gentle stretching and massage. The neck needs care and attention, and any severe pains or debility need medical attention. For some advice about stretching, see appendix 4.

Some favorite home remedies for simple neck stiffness are warm packs, hot showers with gentle stretching of the neck and shoulders, an arnica ointment rubdown after shower, and the warm hands of a friend or body therapist.

Nervous System: See Stress, Memory, and Depression.

Osteoarthritis and the Bones: See Arthritis. The weakening of the bones is a common symptom in aging that can be greatly reduced by three actions: healthful foods (see line of defense 1), regular exercise, and avoidance of harmful foods. Calcium-rich foods include dark leafy greens, nuts and seeds, and whole-grain foods. Kale has more calcium per weight than milk. Excess milk products can be proinflammatory, particularly the milk that we get now from cows raised on corn and antibiotics. Small amounts of cheese, yogurt, and butter are fine. Foods that leach calcium are those that are too acidic or those empty of nutrients: sugar, too much citrus or tomato products, too much coffee, and a diet high in white-flour products. Vitamin D is nourishing for the bones. A little sunshine infuses the body with vitamin D, and vitamin D can be found in fish, grains, and some vegetables. Consult lines of defense 1 through 4.

Performance: Some foods and herbal medicines have the reputation for increasing performance, and this includes athletic, musical, and intellectual. See lines of defense 1 and 2.

Herbal medicines can be helpful. The most well known is Siberian ginseng (also called eleuthero). Other herbal medicines to consider include bacopa, the ginsengs, tribulus, cordyceps, gynostemma, rhodiola, and ashwagandha. There are others, and some very good synergistic formulas, depending on the need and constitution of the person. Consult a health professional knowledgeable about herbal medicine.

Peridontal Disease: See Gum Disease.

PMS (*Premenstrual Syndrome*): A common complaint, particularly with busy modern women who are under a variety of stresses. Common symptoms include cramps, bloating, swollen tender breasts, fatigue, irritability, and changeable moods. Symptoms of PMS can be greatly relieved by stress reduction, stretching, exercise, and good nutrition. Consult the advice under lines of defense 1 and 2.

Many good herbs and vitamins can assist in alleviating this unpleasant condition. For recurrent or intense PMS it is best to see a health practitioner for a complete program. Helpful herbal medicines include dong quai, Saint-John's-wort, vitex, white peony, false unicorn, and black cohosh. Try dandelion leaf tea two to three times a day for fluid retention. Prime nutrients include vitamin B_6, B-complex vitamins, vitamin E, calcium/magnesium, evening primrose oil (1 capsule, 500 mg, once daily), or synergistic formulas with these vitamins and herbs. Also, reduce red meat, sugar, chocolate, coffee, and other stimulants, as well as greasy or cold foods (such as ice cream), and eat plenty of vitamin-rich foods. Saturated fats can be a culprit in PMS, coupled with a deficiency of omega-3 fatty acids. Emotions can be a critical underlying factor, especially suppressed anger or anxiety. Try acupuncture, yoga, therapy, and just plain playfulness.

Dong quai (dang gui) and peony formulas are common in Oriental medicine, or dong quai and bupleurum when discomfort is more of a factor.

Prostate: Problems with the prostate often are a sign of inflammation. A diet rich in saturated fats, alcohol, and sugar can contribute to prostate problems. For some useful advice for preventing prostate problems, consult lines of defense 1 through 4.

Regular checkups are important for men over fifty, especially for those with a family history of cancer or with genitourinary problems. Fifty percent of men over fifty experience some degree of prostatic enlargement. Natural remedies can help incipient prostate problems, the most common of which is prostatic enlargement (BPH). The first signs of this problem include increasingly frequent night urination, difficulty in urinating, or dribbling of urine. Any urinary or prostate problems need to be monitored by a doctor, and BPH should not be self-diagnosed. Therapy for prevention includes a sensible whole-foods diet and reduction of poor-quality fats, meat, and alcohol. Common medicinal herbs include saw palmetto, pygeum, pumpkin seed, nettle root, Asian ginseng, and pipsissewa. First choice is saw palmetto capsules or tablets two to three times daily for two to three months. It is best to include essential fatty acids, vitamins C and E, and zinc in this preventive program. Rich sources of zinc include oysters, wheat bran, whole oatmeal, and pumpkin and sunflower seeds. Drink plenty of good-quality water. Sometimes, when there is not adequate ejaculation, prostate problems can ensue.

Caution: See a physician for urinary retention or blood in the urine.

Psoriasis: This is a complex skin problem that has no easy answers in holistic or conventional medicine. No one knows the cause of psoriasis, indeed if there is one cause. Like eczema, another chronic skin problem, psoriasis presents classic signs of inflammation. A very stubborn condition that can last for many years, psoriasis can be helped by studying the information in lines of defense 1 through 4. Herbalists will often use omega-3 fatty acids and herbs like Oregon grape root, dandelion root, sarsaparilla, and milk thistle, as well as specific dietary advice. In Oriental medicine, psoriasis is related to three factors: liver harmony and ability to detoxify the blood, inflammation in the small intestines, and chronic stress that affects the digestive and nervous systems. The first step in treating this condition is diet and nutrition. The advice offered in lines of defense 1 through 4 can help, but it is best to follow specific guidelines given by a health professional.

Respiratory Problems: See Cough and Sinusitis.

Sciatica: With this condition, nerves down one leg (occasionally both legs) become painful. Numbness, shooting pain, and burning are some of the descriptions of this condition, which is often accompanied by low back pain. Often the cause of sciatica is too much sitting, not enough stretching and exercise, and a lot of stress and tension (for example, indecision about a job change). I have treated hundreds of cases of this common problem. Sometimes it is a good idea to have a medical checkup for any stubborn or long-term pain in the low back and legs, but most of the time, sciatica is caused by a pinched nerve. The referred pain can be anywhere in the leg and can change sporadically. In my experience, sciatica begins with low back muscular tension and an imbalance in the two sides of the low back and hips. One side becomes dominant, the side that manifests the nerve pinch. Acupuncture can be very helpful, as can massage and chiropractic. However, if the treatment does not address the tense trigger points in the hips and low back on the dominant side, the treatment might not work. Stretching can be helpful for treatment and prevention.

Please peruse line of defense 2, as well as appendix 4, stretching.

Sex Drive: Quality sexuality is closely connected to intimacy, affection, mutual respect, and love. However, diminished sex drive can also be a sign of stress, aging, overwork, and lowered vitality. If this is the case, natural alternatives can help considerably, making for a happier, more fulfilled human being. See lines of defense 1 through 3.

Oriental medicine offers a wide array of solutions, including herbal formulas, specialized exercises, and foods. Chinese herbalism has a number of herbs that improve the sex drive. Herbal formulas, however, are generally administered to the individual needs of each patient. In other words, ten people could receive a different formula, a very different attitude than current Western practice where drugs like Viagra are readily prescribed. Viagra's primary effect is to increase blood supply to the penis, and its popularity (and the profit) is indicative of a significant need in the public. Unfortunately, not much attention has been placed on one side of this controversial issue. Little attention is paid to the possible side effects of this drug and related drugs, specifically in long-term use; these could include a burden on the kidneys and liver, possible increase of blood pressure, and strain on the heart.

Herbal medicines to consider with a health professional: maca, ginseng, epimedium, muira puama (Polynesian herb), damiana, and tribulus.

Diminished sex drive can be a warning sign of a more serious underlying disorder that needs medical attention: high blood pressure, obesity, diabetes, and psychological inhibitions.

For more advice, see Male Remedies and Female Remedies in this chapter, as well as Fatigue and Exhaustion. It is unfortunate that in our culture, honest and helpful advice about a healthy sex life is not more readily available, particularly to teenagers.

Sexually Transmitted Diseases (STDs): Besides the advice and treatment by your medical doctor, helpful information can be found in lines of defense 3 and 4. Also, please consult Cleansing in this chapter.

Shingles: Post-hepatic neuralgia (herpes zoster) results in a pain that can linger in some people, particularly the elderly, for months—a distressing condition, to say the least. See lines of defense 1 through 4 for some useful information. Herbs that boost the immune system and lessen inflammation can be helpful. Some tips: Take extra vitamin C and B-complex vitamins as well as omega-3 fatty acids. L-lysine is an amino acid that can help. The beneficial fatty acids can decrease the inflammation that is causing the pain. For those who want to avoid painkillers, try acupuncture. Topically, I also advise Saint-John's-wort lotion or spray. This can relax the painful nerve endings, as well as heal the problem.

Sinusitis: This is a common problem with busy, modern people who are on the go, eat fast foods, and are exposed to urban air. Sinusitis is an inflammation and pain in sinus cavities above the eyes and around the nose, often with postnasal drip or mucus discharge, a difficulty breathing through the nose, as well as local tenderness, pain, and congestion. The common cold or flu or viral or bacterial infections are often involved in sinus problems and often need medical attention. There are remedies that can help in short-term or mild cases: goldenseal (particularly when there is a yellow, thick nasal discharge), echinacea, eyebright or elderberry flower formulas, pau d'arco, astragalus, and ginger. A healing tea includes equal parts of echinacea, goldenseal, and marshmallow leaf. Drink a cup every two to three hours. Also, take garlic and vitamin C internally. Cleaning out the sinuses with a mild saline solution is highly recommended.

An effective home remedy to clear the nasal cavity: Inhale the aromas of herbs like eucalyptus, pine, tea tree oil, or thyme. For those people who suffer from sinus problems, steam inhalation treatment can provide relief. Place the pine, thyme, or eucalyptus tea (or 5 to 8 drops of tea tree oil) into a bowl of hot water, and breathe the fumes with a towel draped over the head to capture the steam. Caution: If there is a serious fever, severe pain, foul-smelling discharge, or a problem in the vicinity of the eyes, seek medical attention.

Long-term sinusitis is a sign of toxic overload and inflammation. Simplify the diet with lean meats, fresh vegetables and fruits, and whole grains, and take an antioxidant formula and essential fatty acids. Drastically reduce white-flour and milk products, which are mucus forming and lead to sinus congestion. To this base program, add the appropriate herbs or herbal formulas.

Also, consult headings under Cough, Lungs, and Immune System. In Oriental medicine, sinus problems are sometimes linked to constipation (see Constipation in this chapter).

Acupressure or acupuncture can help relieve the symptoms of sinusitis. There are key trigger points on either side of the nostrils, under the cheekbones, and right on top of the scalp.

Skin: There are many problems that can afflict the skin: acne, eczema, psoriasis, herpes zoster, and urticaria (hives). Many of these require expert advice. It is important to remember, however, that the skin is an organ of elimination, and some health professionals feel that chronic skin problems are related to problems of inflammation, toxicity, and elimination. See lines of defense 1 through 5. Overloading the liver and blood with poor-quality fats and chemicals is not going to help heal skin problems. Also, the bowels must be functioning well (see Constipation in this chapter).

Some of the best herbal remedies to consider include guggul, pau d'arco, sassafras, red clover, Oregon grape root, and flaxseed or fish oils. Synergistic formulas with burdock are a general herbal strategy for stubborn skin problems with itching and redness. Oregon grape root is another herb with a reputation for healing stubborn skin problems.

Essential fatty acids are an important supplement, as are the plant phytochemicals found in all fresh vegetables and fruits. Some chronic skin problems may involve food allergies: dairy, wheat, peanut butter, and others. Consult an appropriate health professional.

Acne, marked by inflammation of the skin, is a particularly unpleasant skin problem. For those seeking natural treatment to alleviate the symptoms, seek an appropriate health professional, but much of the advice in lines of defense

1, 2, 3, and 4 can be of great help. While acne is often related to hormonal changes in teenagers, it is good to consider that many teenagers consume a proinflammatory diet: particularly saturated fats, sugar, and poor-quality meat.

For dry skin, abrasions, mild burns, and minor rashes, the following external skin-care remedies are suggested: calendula, aloe vera, Saint-John's-wort tincture, olive oil, tea tree oil, or echinacea (cream or lotion). Calendula lotion or ointment is a good all-around remedy for skin health.

Sleeplessness (Insomnia and Restlessness): Very common in people who generally do not get enough good-quality sleep, sleeplessness is most often a sign of excess stress and thinking too much about problems in life. See the advice under line of defense 2. During the deepest part of sleep, the liver sends hormones into the blood to repair and rejuvenate cells throughout the body. For this and other reasons, good-quality sleep is essential for vigor and good health. In many cases of occasional restless nights, the following suggestions can be very helpful: Do not drink stimulants like caffeine drinks three to four hours before going to bed, or at all; engage in vigorous exercise during the day, not just for ten minutes but up to one hour; learn some relaxation exercises with tapes, classes, or books; and do not eat a large meal within four hours of bedtime. Rising late can be counterproductive, as can be naps. Herbal remedies include valerian, California poppy, skullcap, hops, reishi, passionflower, and Saint-John's-wort. Valerian and kava kava formulas are recommended, but for those with liver problems there are restrictions with the very effective herb kava. A soothing passionflower and hops tea (a strong half cup) one hour before retiring, with the rest of the cup next to the bed to be used if needed, can be helpful. Calcium and B vitamins can also relax the nervous system so that the herbal remedies can work better. One Oriental herbal formula is suan zao ren, or take two tablets along with 150 mg of valerian. Suan zao ren calms the nervous system, making sleep more comfortable.

Sore Throat: Most of the common everyday sore throats are due to a localized inflammation caused by some kind of stress. Because bacterial invasions are involved in some sore throats, visit your doctor for sore throats that are accompanied by pain and fever. Also, consider advice under line of defense 3.

For mild, short-term sore throats, try echinacea (as a tea or gargle), andrographis, sage, thyme, echinacea/goldenseal, and pau d'arco. Tea tree lozenges are good. Vitamin C lozenges with zinc and echinacea are a superb combination. Garden sage makes an excellent gargle for sore throats; one can make a tea from the dried herb or buy the extract and add some drops to water. My favorite remedy for simple sore throats is vitamin C and echinacea, three times daily. Also, for scratchy or mild sore throats, try vitamin C or a similar kind of lozenges.

Sports Injuries/Muscle Strain: Localized inflammations initially respond well to ice. For those mild injuries that do not need a medical exam, first apply ice for five to ten minutes, then repeat later in the day. After the pain has subsided a little bit, gently apply arnica ointment. Formulas with boswellia or turmeric are highly recommended for muscle and joint inflammation. Also, see remedies for Arthritis and Tendinitis.

Sports Performance: See Performance.

Stomach: See Indigestion.

Stress: Please consult line of defense 2. Certain foods can aggravate stress, others moderate it: see line of defense 1. Foods rich in omega-3 fatty acids (such as fish, leafy green vegetables, and some nuts) and those abundant in B-complex vitamins (such as eggs and some vegetables) are very helpful. Herbal medicines can also mitigate some of the effects of stress, trauma, and overwork. For generalized stress from overwork or too much exertion, consider one of the following: ginseng (all kinds), ashwagandha, reishi, gynostemma, an antioxidant vitamin formula with herbs and the B vitamins, chamomile, schisandra, he shou wu, morinda, eclipta, muira puama (Polynesian herb), Saint-John's-wort, rehmannia, gotu kola, kava kava, or valerian. Baths with essential oil of rosemary or lavender are very relaxing. For nervous stress, try Saint-John's-wort. For mental/emotional stress, try ashwagandha. For stress to the immune system, astragalus formulas work well. For stress to the whole body, try ginseng and astragalus formulas. See Anxiety and Nervousness, Depression, and Sleeplessness. The famous Oriental herbal formula Rehmannia Six is often used to alleviate stress and can be purchased at quality health food stores.

Stroke: For prevention of stroke, consult Stress, Cleansing, Blood Pressure, and Atherosclerosis, and consult lines of defense 1, 2, 3, and 4. High blood pressure and atherosclerosis are both risk factors in causing strokes. We want to avoid susceptibility to strokes. A stroke is a serious medical condition that occurs when the blood supply to the brain is cut or interrupted, often caused by blood clots, compression, or blood ruptures in the brain. An array of neurological problems can ensue, such as speech and locomotion problems. If you have suffered from a stroke, some natural methods can help considerably, with professional advice. Recommended are certain kinds of foods and herbs, such as dan shen (a common Oriental herb), ginkgo, hawthorn, and grapeseed extract. For specific foods that can help prevent stroke, consult line of defense 1.

Tendinitis: This is inflammation of the tendons due to injury, most commonly strain, such as playing too much tennis (tennis elbow).

Once the tendon has been strained, which causes the pain, one must look after the area of injury and not overuse it. Otherwise, the tendon will not heal. The first thing to do is put ice on it.

To reduce pain, try a ginger compress made from fresh ginger. Herbs that help are ginger, bromelain, and boswellia.

Arnica ointment, rubbed gently into and around the area every day, will soothe and help reduce swelling. Follow the pain down the arm toward the wrist and massage this line. There is always a line of muscular tension related to tendinitis. Finding this and releasing it sometimes can be the cure.

For stubborn cases, consult lines of defense 1 through 3 and see an acupuncturist.

Ulcerative Colitis: This is a potentially serious medical problem that requires medical attention. If seeking alternatives to conventional medicine, which mostly offers drug therapy, see an expert in natural medicine. The symptoms of this problem are aggravated, even caused by, underlying stress and inflammation in the intestines. A holistic approach involving diet, stress management, and herbal medicines is a sensible strategy. See lines of defense 1 through 4. Many herbs are healthy for the intestines, and these are always combined with a healthy diet. Some herbs to consider include flaxseeds, peppermint, chamomile, boswellia, acidophilus (probiotics), and turmeric. Also, see Irritable Bowel Syndrome and Indigestion. See probiotics in appendix 2.

Ulcers: Peptic ulcers are internal sores (lesions) that occur as a result of multiple stresses. Bacteria, underlying inflammation, and stress are often major causes of ulcers. See line of defense 1 for an overview of diet. Consult line of defense 2 for advice about stress reduction and line of defense 3 for overview of detoxification.

The lining of the stomach is damaged when the stomach is unable to release protective mucus secretion. To prevent ulcers, try licorice, cabbage juice, goldenseal, peppermint, or chamomile tea, but for active ulcers, see a professional. See Indigestion.

Urinary Tract Infections (UTIs): Underlying inflammation and stress can lead to predisposition to urinary tract infections. Though often caused by bacteria, the germs are only taking advantage of an unhealthy ecology. See a health professional for advice. There are times when antibiotics could be needed. Preventive measures can help considerably. Consult lines of defense 2 and 3. Drink plenty of water. Herbal medicines to consider for prevention include barberry, bearberry (uva ursi), goldenseal, juniper, and celery seed. Cranberry juice cleans the bladder, but it is best to use organic juice that has no sugar. Drink small amounts mixed with water several times daily. Synergistic bladder formulas are a good way to go, and these can be used as directed several times daily for a few days. Avoid sweets, sugars, poor-quality fats, and excess rich carbohydrates.

Caution: Any pain, blood in, or restriction of urine requires prompt medical attention.

Urticaria: Hives. See Skin.

Vaginal Discharges: This is another classic sign of inflammation and toxification. For general information about prevention, consult lines of defense 3 and 4. These discharges are often due to proliferation of yeast infection with itching, offensive odor, mild inflammation, and white to yellow discharge. Excess sugars, sweet drinks, dairy products, cold foods, fried foods, and junk food can make a woman prone to discharges. Essential oils of chamomile, tea tree, or lavender (8 drops) can be stirred into warm bath water for a soothing, cleansing bath. Certain soaps, tampons, nylon underwear, tight polyester clothing, swimming pool water, and scented toilet papers may irritate the vaginal area. Prolonged use of antibiotics and other drugs can make a woman prone to vaginal infections. Herbs that are good for douches include pau d'arco, calendula, and goldenseal. Herbal medicines that are effective are pau d'arco, goldenseal, pulsatilla (homeopathic), echinacea, garlic, and acidophilus. For external use, try calendula or Saint-John's-wort tincture or lotion.

Caution: Any unusual vaginal discharge needs a medical examination.

Veins: Varicose veins are a condition that produces bulging, bluish veins and often results from poor circulation due to lack of exercise, sedentary lifestyle (sitting on your butt), and faulty diet—the white-food diet. See lines of defense 1 through 3. To improve circulation, increase exercise, lose weight if you are overweight, move your bowels regularly, and eat plenty of whole grains, fruits, and vegetables. Herbs that help include gotu kola, ginseng, ginkgo, horse chestnut, and bilberry. Topically, horse chestnut, witch hazel, or butcher's broom work well. Foods rich in vitamins C and E are particularly recommended, including carrots, celery, leafy green vegetables, beans, peas, apples, and nuts.

Viral Infections: See Flu. Most viruses become active only when the system is out of balance, overstressed, and weak. See lines of defense 1 and 5. If a viral infection is suspected, medical attention should be sought. Specific herbs include echinacea, goldenseal, Saint-John's-wort flower-top tea, olive leaf extract, red clover, cedar, schisandra, lemon balm, and osha. Herbal antiviral formulas can be purchased, as well as excellent immune-boosting combinations. Viral infections are more potent when inflammation and toxification are present (see lines of defense 3 and 4). We can protect ourselves from susceptibility to viral infections with natural health methods and by avoiding the panic that often afflicts the general public.

Vision: See Eyes.

Weight Loss: Losing weight is not easy. Fast-food culture surrounds us, and fast foods have a certain comfort value: fatty, greasy, and sweet. We become habituated to these comfort foods. Furthermore, being overweight is an inflammatory condition that makes us more lethargic (and worse yet, apathetic). See lines of defense 1 through 4. Finally, there is the

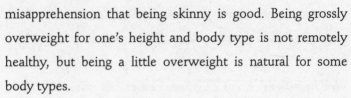

misapprehension that being skinny is good. Being grossly overweight for one's height and body type is not remotely healthy, but being a little overweight is natural for some body types.

Millions of dollars are made every year on programs to lose weight—books, diets, tapes—and most of it is a waste of time and money. Some of the specialized diets could even be harmful, and much of the time the weight comes back. Dr. Andrew Weil once said that there are two words that cover weight loss: *Eat less.* I think there are four words: *Eat less, exercise more.* Obesity is a problem of civilization: too much fatty and sugary foods around to tempt us. Being too sedentary is also a problem of civilization. People go from their car, to their office, to their television chair, and then to bed. And to top it off, their diet is the rich white-food diet that has been mentioned many times in this book: see line of defense 1. This sluggish and devitalizing diet creates real obstacles to better health and energy. Stress and tension are factors that can force us to eat excessively and impulsively (consult line of defense 2).

To lose weight it is important to set clear goals. Write them down. Be specific. List what you are going to do; enlist your friends and family to support you. Also, be realistic, several pounds a month, and sometimes we will slip, but the goals extend over three to twelve months, even longer. Be passionate about achieving your goals. No one wants to know the bottom line in losing weight. There are two: Exercise so that you sweat, and consume your cheap calories, especially sugar and sugary foods (especially candy, cookies, muffins, and sweets) and fatty, greasy foods. Choose an exercise that you like; for some, it is better to exercise with other people. Sweating is a sign that you are burning off calories.

When you are overweight and you really want to lose the weight, it is best to follow a weight-loss program for several months. Once again, one can do it with other people—this can help. However, it is important to realize that body types respond better to different diets (see line of defense 1). Eating less carbohydrates and sugary foods is the key here, and adding sufficient protein and low-starch vegetables. Avoiding all sugary foods and white-flour products is a huge step forward. A high-protein diet has helped some people, but this would not be recommended for a long time.

Eating a little less than you need is a good way to live a long life.

Do the heavily advertised weight-loss pills help? Many of them can be harmful in the long run. However, there are some natural supplements that can be of some assistance, if the main program is followed: healthy diet and more exercise. The mineral chromium has been known to help some people. Take as directed. High fiber can provide bulk, decrease calories and appetite, and cleanse the system. A nutritional supplement called 5-HTP has shown some positive results. Herbal medicines that can help in various ways (see a qualified herbalist) include Saint-John's-wort, the ginsengs, gynostemma, and dandelion root. Triphala, a standby in Ayurvedic medicine, is a general tonic and cleanser that can help some people using diet and exercise. Food supplements like green foods can supply energy and a range of nutrients.

The advertising world convinces us that we have to be thin like the models in the magazines. Most of us will never be five feet, eleven inches with a weight of 110 pounds. Some of us would not want to look like this. Some of us were born stocky and short, chunky or round. Be proud of what we are. And remember the advice of my good friend Dennis: Have more sex. It is a good way to consume calories.

CHAPTER 5

Health Promotion and Longevity

WE ALL WANT TO BE IN OPTIMAL HEALTH IN OUR DAY-TO-DAY
lives, and we would like to ensure that we live long and pro-
ductive lives. All of us hope that our last years are not burdened by poor health, pain, and stiffness. All the information
presented in this book will help people defend their health,
increase their energy, and promote a long life.

Struggling against the many stresses in life is an ongoing
and rewarding challenge. As discussed in chapter 2, the various
and prolonged stresses of life can wear us down, overtax the
liver and other organs, and create conditions of inflammation
and disease. Information related in this book about nutrition,

stress reduction, and exercise will ensure that our struggle will succeed. By reducing toxification and inflammation we can ensure better health and less disease.

In this book and many other health books on the market, we are deluged by information and facts. In our society, there are many complex terms, disease names, and countless advice about drugs, vitamins, and other solutions to health problems. There are different diets that all claim to be the best. We could throw up our hands and run away from a more proactive attitude toward health promotion. If the readers of this book go away with anything, I would hope they have understood several basic facts about health promotion.

✳ The importance of healthy fats in our daily diet and reduction of poor-quality fats. This would also include reduction of the white-food diet. Omega-3 fatty acids have many important roles in maintaining health of the heart, nerves, and brain. Review line of defense 1 in chapter 3. In the past sixty years, the American diet has switched to proinflammatory fats, causing a new wave of ill health and disease predisposition.

✳ The importance of a variety of antioxidants in our diet. As discussed in chapter 2, antioxidants are constituents of fruits and vegetables that reduce stress in the body, counteract toxins, and prevent disease. We should eat a variety of antioxidant-rich food every day, especially leafy greens, root vegetables like carrots, and fruits like apples. And conversely, we need to reduce foods that inhibit the action of these antioxidants. We need to avoid the proinflammatory diet (see lines of defense 1 and 4).

✻ The importance of a variety of exercises in our daily lives, from simple walking to stretching to working out. In this book, exercise signifies more than sports activity, more than moving the body in walking or swimming; it means moving the heart and mind and body. Our minds need exercise through reading, pondering, and playing. Our hearts need exercise with friendship, creative activities, music, and art.

We need to engage the whole body—the physical, emotional, and mental—in a variety of ways. It is especially good when you love the exercise of your choice. I see people dancing passionately, or skating, or yoga—it feels good. Spending time on our bodies, not for vanity but for sensible care, is one of our best investments. An hour a day for the body tune-up is an investment in optimal health and longevity.

Our attitudes and feelings affect our bodies, health, and longevity. For years I have studied the habits and attitudes of healthy seniors, people in their eighties and nineties. Some of these people have come to me as patients. Some of these elders are truly remarkable people, busy, active, and creative. They have maintained exercise of their whole being into their twilight years, and often they seem younger than people twenty years younger. They are not particularly fussy about foods, yet they have eaten a good, sensible, balanced diet with a minimum of fast foods. They have engaged their minds in games, books, friends, and projects. Most often they are independent, suspicious of taking too many medications, and they certainly display a feisty side. Always, they have a good circle of friends and creative activities. They are an inspiration to us all.

I knew a truly incredible man of ninety-nine who was still teaching math part time at a prestigious university. One lady in her mid-nineties maintained a whole array of friends of all ages. One of my patients, who is ninety-two, has swum three times a week for years. She is slender and active, sings in a group, and displays a great sense of humor. An acceptance of what life gives us, gratefulness for this body, and a sense of humor about all the contradictions and disappointments are a wonderful triad of traits.

Sadly our culture often puts the elderly into homes where sometimes the opportunities are fewer. In nursing homes, I have seen them grossly overmedicated. Much is said about good genes and longevity, and there is truth in this, but one can also see that a life well lived, with gusto and variety, is the greatest gift of all.

Our health is a precious gift and our body a remarkable machine. We need to respect and support this body for its remarkable talents and gifts. We need to give it a tune-up several times a week: playtime, relaxation, deep relaxation, meditation, exercise, and affection. We do need to work to defend our health. Disease and discomfort will be less, and the rewards are many.

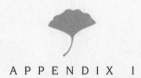

Health Tips to Incorporate into Life

＊ Eating less than we need is one of the keys to longevity. Stuffing oneself to capacity at every meal is a burden on the whole body. Thank goodness that Thanksgiving comes only once a year.

＊ Drink adequate water each day, up to eight glasses, less if drinking tea or coffee. Also, listen to the needs of your body: Some people drink *too* much water!

＊ Every culture has appreciated and benefited from herbal teas: boiled water infused with herbs or an herb. Many of these teas contain nutrients and antioxidants that prevent disease, inflammation, and pain. Common teas include green, black, and chamomile.

❋ Lemon juice from real lemons is particularly healthful, just half a glass once in a while, more when tired or overtaxed. Lemon juice is good for the liver and detoxification.

❋ Olive oil is the best. It is best cold-pressed and virgin with a slightly dark coloring.

❋ Avoid partially hydrogenated oils as much as possible. They are in margarine, many commercial salad dressings, fried foods, and hidden in many processed foods like potato chips.

❋ Beware of many fast foods. Some are not only loaded with calories but also potentially harmful saturated and trans fats. One serving of a hamburger, French fries, and a fancy coffee drink can have more than your weekly allowance of saturated fats.

❋ Enjoy fresh air and sunshine every day if possible, but not too much sun and wear some protection. Sunlight is abundant in life energy. It is the source of heat, light, and energy on our planet.

❋ Enjoy nature: trees, flowers, lakes, forests, and parks. They are abundant in vitality that enriches our bodies. Exercise every day!

❋ Enjoy food and eating. The French are a good example of a culture that has made a spectacular art of eating, and they don't feel much guilt about their "sinful" pleasures. Because of the quality of their diet—a variety of tasty and healthy foods—they are less prone to the many inflammatory diseases that afflict Americans.

✳ Enjoy small amounts of alcohol several times a week. Wine is rich in healthful antioxidants. Good, well-made beer is an herbal beverage. Do not follow this advice if it is contrary to your medical needs or if you have an addiction to alcohol.

✳ Consume a small amount of fermented food weekly— yogurt, sauerkraut, miso, kefir, wine, certain cheeses—and consider using acidophilus and related supplements occasionally. These contain healthful substances for general health. See appendix 2.

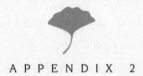

APPENDIX 2

The Best Hits of the Supplements

Supplements are products that we take in addition to our daily diet. Our daily food is the foundation and for the most part offers us all we need. However, because of the excess stress and chemicals of modern life, we can do with a boost.

✳ Vitamins and minerals, often found in capsules or tablets. Many people take a multivitamin daily, perfectly adequate for most. Some people also add a calcium and magnesium supplement. Also recommended are specialized antioxidant formulas, with vitamins A, C, and E, zinc, selenium, and other constituents. I recommend these during times of stress or during the cold season.

❋ Concentrated food supplements are often found in powder or pills. For example, many companies market excellent green food supplements that you add to water or milk and stir. Spirulina is a highly concentrated green food supplement extraordinarily rich in a variety of nutrients. Because such supplements are less processed and more absorbable, in some ways I prefer them to a daily vitamin.

❋ Herbal supplements are whole-food medicines with specific health benefits. I find herbs to be a bridge between drug therapy and food therapy. Safer than medical drugs, they can be used for general health purposes and with professional guidance for treatment of disease. See appendix 3.

❋ Probiotics are good for the digestion and general health. We hear a lot about antibiotics in America, but little about probiotics, the beneficial bacteria that support health and vigor.

Fermented and sour foods such as yogurt, buttermilk, kefir, miso, sauerkraut, and some cheeses contain acidophilus or other beneficial microorganisms that are healthy for the intestines and the whole body. These microorganisms help to promote the healthy ecology of the intestines where thousands of bacteria work to maintain health. Many of these good guys flourish in our own bodies, their chief factory being the intestines, where they assist in the digestive processes and inhibit the proliferation of pathogenic organisms. Lactobacillus and bifidus are among the chief beneficial bacteria that thrive in our guts. Modern processed diet, excess antibiotics, oral contraceptives, aspirin, steroids, and excess sugar are among the culprits that disturb the ecology of the intestines, resulting in chronic bowel problems, decreased resistance to disease, and lowered energy levels. Bloating, gas, and irritable bowels are some of the common symptoms attributable to depletion of these friendly bacteria. Even more critical is the poor assimilation of foods and general toxic overload, the groundwork for many diseases.

Probiotics may be useful for health problems including cancer, rapid aging, arthritis, diarrhea, high cholesterol, systemic candida albicans, vaginal yeast infections, bladder infections, and constipation; and during chemotherapy and radiation. When antibiotics are used or abused, acidophilus or related products should be consumed regularly.

DAILY SUPPLEMENTS: WHAT TO TAKE

For the purpose of general health I recommend the following, although they should not all be taken at once, or all the time. In fact, people sometimes can overindulge in supplements, a whole squadron of vitamin bottles. If we eat well, as recommended in line of defense 1, there is little or no need for any supplementation.

Food Facts

Fermented milk goes by many names around the world. Traditional diets have always valued the benefit of these and other fermented foods. Fermented milk owes its potency to a large family of bacteria called lactobacillus (L.bifidus is another major one). When mixed into milk, these bacteria proliferate and cause the milk to ferment and curdle, which results in the sour taste. The result is a remarkable change in the chemical composition of the milk, a potent health-producing super food. Cheeses, sour milks, yogurts, as well as certain fermented vegetables (cabbage, soybeans, and others) can contain these healthful properties. Many of these products, however, lose their potency if they are not fresh or properly made—and this includes freeze-dried acidophilus capsules. Homemade yogurt, sour milk, and fermented cabbage are good sources of lactobacillus.

Excess antibiotics (and certain other prescription drugs), chlorinated water, and a diet high in meat products can disturb the ecology of the intestines and thus diminish the healthful lactobacilli. A diet low in vegetables, fruits, and fiber can also upset the ecology of the intestine, leading to many serious health problems.

Other common sources of fermented foods: In Indonesia, tempeh, a delicious soybean product, is very popular. In China, Japan, and other Asian countries, fermented cabbage and miso are healthful fermented foods.

What should I buy? Some products are not so valuable so it is best to shop carefully. Products must contain L. acidophilus and/or B. bifidum in a quality preparation that can be absorbed and utilized by the body. Refrigeration is often necessary, but some products do not have to be refrigerated until the bottle has been opened. Many people now realize that when taking antibiotics, it is good to ingest extra acidophilus, either as a supplement or food. Do not take the antibiotics at the same time. Not all yogurts are created equal; most supermarket yogurts are not true fermented foods. Purchase yogurt that has been naturally fermented and not adulterated by sugar and preservatives.

* Daily multivitamin. This is the simplest and most sensible addition to a healthful daily diet.
* An omega-3 fatty acid supplement. One blend I like is capsules with flaxseed and borage seed oil. Some people pre-

cause, taken in excess this can result in vitamin A toxicity. Liquid flaxseed oil, which needs refrigeration, is cheaper than the capsules. I especially recommend omega-3 supplementation for anyone with any inflammatory syndrome. See line of defense 4.

❋ Vitamin E, preferably the natural version, is a powerful antioxidant with antinflammatory properties. The natural version is designated by a d, as in d-tocopherol.

❋ Vitamin C. I prefer the vitamin C that also contains bioflavonoids. In nature, vitamin C is related to bioflavonoids, also potent antioxidants. A typical dose would be 500 mg daily.

❋ Use kitchen herbs and spices in your cooking. Herbs like garlic, rosemary, turmeric, pepper, and basil have multiple therapeutic properties—detoxifying and anti-inflammatory.

❋ Milk thistle, dandelion root, and schisandra are medicinal herbs that are beneficial to the liver and detoxification. See appendix 3.

❋ Siberian ginseng is good for energy. Astragalus is good for the immune system. Asian ginseng is good for people over forty with tiredness and lack of zip. See appendix 3.

❋ Alpha lipoic acid, a natural supplement that has antioxidant properties.

Longevity: The Short List

Some foods and supplements that could help to promote longevity and vigor:

* A multivitamin
* Omega-3 fatty acids
* The phytochemicals in many fruits and vegetables, especially green leafy vegetables, nuts like walnuts and almonds, fish, herbs and spices like rosemary, coriander, turmeric, and basil
* Beans, such as pinto or black, are rich in fiber and vitamins
* Longevity herbs—see discussion in chapter 3—include reishi mushroom, ginseng, and gotu kola

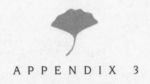

APPENDIX 3

Medicinal Plants

This appendix is a primer to the major medicinal plants for detoxification and immune enhancement. Herbs are safe, natural medicines, good for health promotion, energy, and immune support. There are no medical drugs that can do what herbal medicines can do, and for the most part herbal medicines are much safer than pharmaceutical drugs. (Conversely, synthetic drugs can accomplish what herbs cannot.) *Herbal medicines exist in a bridge between healthful foods and medical drugs, and for this reason hold a special place in medicine.* I will list some of the best overall herbs for fulfilling the purposes of this book:

health promotion and disease prevention. Furthermore, some of these herbs can support the all-important detoxification of the body. See line of defense 3. All the following herbs have a history of use that goes back thousands of years, and without exception all of them have had extensive scientific testing and clinical use.

ASTRAGALUS: One of the best all-around herbs to boost the immune system and energy. A very famous Oriental herb, astragalus is a truly excellent healing herb that is very safe. It is often used with synergistic herbs like licorice, ginger, and ginseng. Astragalus formulas are rampant in the Orient, and it is probably the best single herb for immune enhancement.

CHAMOMILE: Relaxes the stomach and nerves. To benefit from chamomile, which has numerous therapeutic properties, drink a strong brew. Brew two bags in hot water for at least five minutes and then drink lukewarm several times daily when needed. It can also be found in capsules, liquid extracts, and tablets, often with herbs that also benefit digestion. Chamomile is a major home remedy in Europe.

DONG QUAI: This famous Oriental herb (also spelled dang gui) is a root medicine that vitalizes the blood. It is nourishing for female health, perhaps the best overall tonic for the female body. Also see Female Remedies in chapter 4. Most often it is used alone or in formulas for menstrual difficulties, pain, and menopausal symptoms. It can be taken in capsules several times daily for more than a few weeks.

ECHINACEA: One of the best general herbs for short-term use to boost the immune system; for simple sore throats, colds, swollen glands, and flu. Often taken with elderberry and vitamin C for best advantage. Echinacea is found in liquid extract (good for mixing with water and gargling), capsules, and tablets and is found in formulas with goldenseal or elderberry. Goldenseal and echinacea can be taken three times daily for up to ten days to deter germs.

ELDERBERRY: The liquid extract, tablet, or capsule is a good immune booster and often used during cold and flu season. This very gentle herb is excellent for children. It is sometimes alternated or taken with echinacea.

FISH OIL CAPSULES AND LIQUID: One of my favorite supplements and highly recommended for many people. See Flaxseed for health benefits. Caution, however, with cod liver oil: While healthy for the short term, cod liver oil can deliver too much vitamin A if overused, which is toxic.

FLAXSEED: Flaxseed oil is rich in healthy fats that are good for the brain, blood vessels, and nervous system. The omega-3 fatty acids reduce inflammation (see line of defense 1) and can improve mobility. They are also good for moods, brain functions, and the heart. In health benefits, they are similar to fish oil supplements. Please take these supplements as recommended on the label. They will do little good if not taken regularly for several months.

GARLIC: A pharmacy in itself, garlic inhibits germs, boosts the immune system, and thins the blood. Garlic can be consumed raw (a tough route but effective) when a clove is chopped up and mixed with a little bread and olive oil. It is also available in capsules and tablets—take as recommended for a few days, or as suggested.

GINSENG, ASIAN: Asian ginseng is best for those over forty, and good for general health and energy. Shop carefully—ginseng supplements can vary in quality. Ginseng is the godfather of Oriental herbs because it is the premiere adaptogen, an herb that supports the whole body. Moderate restrictions exist with ginseng. See below.

GINSENG, SIBERIAN: The best all-around adaptogen and tonic. Safe and relatively inexpensive. Siberian ginseng is one of the best medicines to take during any time of stress or overwork.

It is available in liquid extract, capsules, and tablets, and some companies make a standardized product. This herb is fine to take several times daily for a few weeks, but if you are taking any long-term prescription drugs, consult an herbal specialist or physician before using it.

GOLDENSEAL: The famous American Indian herb that helps the body to detoxify, particularly from conditions that create inflammation and mucus. This herb has important anti-inflammatory properties and inhibits many noxious germs. It is always taken for the short term, up to ten days, and often with echinacea. Goldenseal should be avoided by pregnant or nursing women, unless instructed by an herbal specialist. Some restrictions exist for those taking goldenseal with medical drugs—consult your health professional. Goldenseal is better taken in capsules or tablets and is a bitter-tasting herb, the source of its medicinal power.

GREEN TEA: An antioxidant beverage that also supports the immune system. A good tea to consume regularly, green tea is loaded with phytochemicals that support the body in a variety of ways. Green tea is said to help prevent cancer and other degenerative diseases and has been the subject of numerous scientific studies. Black tea is similar but not quite as healthful.

HAWTHORN BERRY: This famous European herbal medicine is rich in nutrients and phytochemicals that are good for the blood vessels and heart. It is found in capsules, tablets, standardized extracts, and synergistic herbal formulas that support the cardiovascular system.

MILK THISTLE: Heals the liver and is good for anyone who has abused their liver with drugs, chemicals, and tension. Milk thistle is one of the best herbal medicines for modern people, along with schisandra. This herb can be found in synergistic formulas (with herbs that enhance its detoxifying properties) or by itself in capsules, tablets, and liquid extracts. This is a very benign herb and has few cautions and restrictions. Some practitioners prefer standardized milk thistle products. These can be taken as recommended, often two to three tablets every day for several weeks.

MUSHROOMS: Medicinal mushrooms have an ancient use in the Orient. They are excellent natural medicines for the immune and nervous systems and have been proven to dramatically boost immune factors. Several key medicinal mushrooms include maitake, which is used in Japan as a cancer preventative; shiitake, the common culinary mushroom; and the legendary reishi, the mushroom of longevity. For overall health benefits and longevity, I recommend a blend of the best medicinal mushrooms—one of the best natural medicines for overall health. Mushroom medicines can be found in natural pharmacies in tablets, capsules, and standardized extracts. Unless you are allergic to mushrooms, they are a very benign medicine with few restrictions or cautions. Like ginseng, mushroom medicines are generally considered a gentle tonic to the whole body.

PEPPERMINT: One of the great home remedies, along with echinacea and chamomile. It can be taken in synergistic formulas, in tablets, liquid extracts, and most commonly as a tea. This is one of the great antispasmodics of the plant kingdom, especially beneficial for the stomach and digestive system: gas, bloating, and aching. When needed, drink a strong brew several times daily for a few days.

SCHISANDRA: Protects the liver from pollutants and helps to heal damaged livers. This famous Oriental herb is one of the best herbs for detoxification. It is very safe and has been researched extensively. It is now found in most natural pharmacies, alone or in synergistic formulas. Take as recommended, often 2 to 3 capsules twice daily for up to several months.

TURMERIC: Reduces inflammation and supports the liver. This is the same as the famous kitchen spice, which can be taken as a supplement as a capsule or tablet. In India, turmeric is one of the great medicines for prevention of cancer and other degenerative diseases. Turmeric natural medicines can be taken as recommended, often twice daily for several months.

CONCLUSION

When you need to take herbs, follow directions and take them regularly for a few days, sometimes twice daily. These are not fast-acting medicines. They are absorbed into the body more like a food and take a little time for their action to influence the body.

CAUTIONS

Herbal medicines, while much safer than synthetic drugs, do have some cautions. Remember, there are poisonous plants in the plant kingdom, but these are *not* available as herbal remedies. Abuse and overuse of concentrated modern preparations of herbs produce almost all the bad press about herbs: for example, the abuse of the valuable Oriental herb ephedra by athletes and weight-loss clients. Ephedra, which is now banned in this country, has been used in its natural form for hundreds of years in the Orient. Nursing or pregnant women should consult an expert before using medicinal doses of any herbs or other plant remedy. Some herbs interact with medical drugs, and some people with long-term medical conditions like high blood pressure, autoimmune diseases, heart disease, and cancer should not take herbs. The best general rule: If you are taking long-term prescription drugs, consult your physician or appropriate health professional before adding medicinal herbs to your regimen.

Used with care and common sense, herbs are safe and effective. I have been using them professionally for twenty-five years and have never had a problem. People have used herbs medicinally for thousands of years, and in many ways they are the perfect support for health promotion.

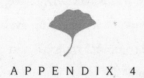

APPENDIX 4

Body Tune-Up and Stretching

WE CAN ALL BENEFIT FROM DAILY STRETCHING, INCLUDING A simple routine that can be added to your body tune-up program. Keeping the body limber and relaxed creates more energy and enjoyment in life. Daily stretching, even for ten minutes a day, is a great way to tune up the body and keep it limber and fit. One of the facts of aging poorly is stiffening joints and lack of suppleness.

Stretching is something we all do instinctively. Bending forward or twisting when we get out of a chair, arching back or forward when we get out of bed, or turning our necks at the end of a long day. We do little stretches here and there.

Our animal friends do this as well. Cats, known for their poise and grace, stretch regularly. We instinctively want to stretch because all our joints and muscles want to be more supple and relaxed. Sitting too much and daily tensions contribute to subtle tensions and stagnations in sections of the body: Particularly vulnerable are the neck and shoulders, low back and hips, and hands and wrists. We have key muscles and joints that should be limbered up every day, particularly for those sitting at computer stations or in cars.

Key joints include the wrists, shoulders, neck, hips, waist, ankles, and knees, as well as the toe and finger joints. Most of the time we don't realize how stiff these joints can be.

Each of these joints can be stretched in a daily whole-body routine, which can take less than fifteen minutes. Or one can do part of it—say the wrists, shoulders, and neck—in the morning, and the lower body in the evening.

For the most part, stretching is safe, gentle, and relaxing and contributes to the whole body tune-up.

PRECAUTIONS

Do not cause pain when stretching. Pain is not gain. If you are doing a simple shoulder roll and it hurts, modify it or see a professional.

Do stretches slowly, repeat up to ten to fifteen times, and

do not rush or overdo it. This is a time of relaxation to tune up your body. Take time to listen to the needs of your body.

Do not stretch if you have injured yourself. First see a doctor or physical therapist for advice.

There are several good books on stretching. *Stretching* by Bob Andersen is one. It is a very good idea to take a class at a local gym or health center, or go to a yoga studio.

There are four basic positions that we can stretch from: standing, lying down on your stomach, lying down on your back, and sitting.

Stretch the whole body. One of the best routines is to stand and gently stretch fingers, wrists, arms and shoulders, and the neck. For example, turn the wrists in slow circles, squeeze and release the fingers, and gently turn the head from left to right several times. Four or five stretches can then be done lying on one's back. For example, raising the knees up to chest one at a time, and doing ten repetitions.

It is important to remember to stretch even the little joints. The feet, toes, and ankles can be stretched. Often people carry tension in their feet and toes. For example, one can lie on one's back and turn the ankles in circles up to ten times, and then stretch out the toes as far as they will go, and then squeeze the toes as one can clench and release one's fingers. All the minor and major joints can then be limbered and tuned up.

One key area not to forget is the waist and lower back. One of the best stretches is to lie down on one's back and then sit up in that position and almost touch one's toes with your fingers. Repeat several times.

One other kind of stretch I always tell my patients is the twist: From a standing position, twist to the left slowly with shoulders and neck and then to the right, up to ten times. Twist as far as one can (no pain!), with one's head and shoulders as if trying to look behind.

Turning on music can make stretching more fun. And if you don't have a slippery shower or bath, a little stretching can be done under hot water. Try incorporating the life-promoting whole body stretch into your life, several times a week, which includes the repetitive and gentle stretching of all the major joints and muscles of the body. Dancing to your favorite music in the living room can accomplish the same goal.

Other forms of good exercise which limber up the body: tai chi, chi kung (Oriental energy practices), basketball, baseball, skating, golf, swimming, bicycling, skiing, and brisk walking.

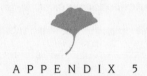

Food Is Our Best Medicine:
Foods to Avoid

FOOD IS OUR BEST MEDICINE, A THEME THAT HAS RESOUNDED throughout history from the age of the ancient Greeks to modern times. Sadly, however, this theme has evaded the modern Western world, that is, until very recently. Except for a minority of nutritionists, alternative medicine practitioners, and doctors, the medical profession has largely overlooked this fundamental fact. The nutritional facts of this book are now supported by many prominent studies. However, one source that has been completely overlooked in the past sixty years is the research of Dr. Weston Price. Dr. Price was very fortunate to visit people in remote areas of the world who

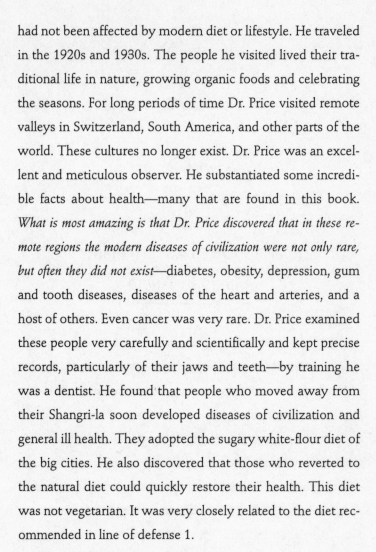

had not been affected by modern diet or lifestyle. He traveled in the 1920s and 1930s. The people he visited lived their traditional life in nature, growing organic foods and celebrating the seasons. For long periods of time Dr. Price visited remote valleys in Switzerland, South America, and other parts of the world. These cultures no longer exist. Dr. Price was an excellent and meticulous observer. He substantiated some incredible facts about health—many that are found in this book. *What is most amazing is that Dr. Price discovered that in these remote regions the modern diseases of civilization were not only rare, but often they did not exist*—diabetes, obesity, depression, gum and tooth diseases, diseases of the heart and arteries, and a host of others. Even cancer was very rare. Dr. Price examined these people very carefully and scientifically and kept precise records, particularly of their jaws and teeth—by training he was a dentist. He found that people who moved away from their Shangri-la soon developed diseases of civilization and general ill health. They adopted the sugary white-flour diet of the big cities. He also discovered that those who reverted to the natural diet could quickly restore their health. This diet was not vegetarian. It was very closely related to the diet recommended in line of defense 1.

What Dr. Price did not find, even in many urban centers of the world, at that time were people who regularly consumed foods like the ones listed below.

FOODS TO WATCH OUT FOR

Many tasty and common foods in American fast-food culture are silent killers. One needs to shop shrewdly, read labels, and be extra cautious with many processed snack foods and fast-foods restaurants. In supermarkets, you can ring the store, mostly shopping in the vegetable and fruit section, in the fish and meat market, and in the dairy section, skipping much of what is in the middle aisles. Read the labels: Especially watch out for hidden sugar, excess salt, and saturated fats. Remember that 2,000 calories a day is sufficient for most people. As we can see from the following examples, single fast-food items—which are sometimes eaten between meals—offer up to half of our needed daily calories. Also, when a packet labels the fat contents: Over 5 grams per serving is getting steep, 20 grams is perverse, especially when 70 percent of that is saturated fats. Furthermore, some of the products that might seem healthier, like whole-grain crackers, can be bogus whole grain loaded with salt and fats.

Here are some shocking examples from a nutrition action healthletter (published by the Center for Science in the Public Interest in Washington, D.C., 2003).

ARTERY CRUST: According to the label, Pepperidge Farm's Flaky Crust Chicken Pot Pie has 450 calories and 7 grams of fat. But look again. Those numbers are for *half* the pie. Eat the entire pie, as most people do, and you're talking 900 calories and 14 grams of saturated fat. Then add the 13 grams of hidden trans fat (which comes from the partially hydrogenated vegetable shortening) in each pie and you're up to 27 grams of artery-clogging fat—that's more than a day's allotment.

BAGELS IN DISGUISE: It's not the bagels in McDonald's Bagel Breakfast Sandwiches that will get you in trouble—it's the fillings. The worst is the Spanish Omelette, with 710 calories and more than half of your daily quota of fat, cholesterol, and salt. To your arteries, that looks like an Egg McMuffin plus a Sausage Biscuit. If you want to have breakfast under the Golden Arches, try the Fruit'n Yogurt Parfait with low-fat milk or orange juice instead.

OUT IN LEFT FIELD: No one expects a Mrs. Field's cookie to be good for you, but who would guess that a single Mrs. Field's Milk Chocolate and Walnuts cookie has more than 300 calories and as much saturated fat as a 12-ounce sirloin steak? It's also got 6 teaspoons of sugar.

CORONARY KING: Burger King makes some of the worst French fries you can buy. A King Size order packs 600 calories and three quarters of your daily maximum for heart-unhealthy fat.

Bowel Wow: Lay's WOW! Potato chips, like Fat-free Pringles, are fried in Olean (Olestra), the indigestible fat substitute. Olean doesn't provide any calories, but in many people it causes gastrointestinal distress. Some people suffer from such severe cramps and diarrhea that they have to go to the emergency room. Olean also reduces the body's absorption of carotenoids.

Some especially blatant examples, the above offers a short glimpse into the food industry. What are people on the run going to do? Most people complain, "I am just too busy to go shopping twice a week for healthy food and to do my own cooking." Please consult line of defense 1 for some easy tips. It's easy to start the day well and healthy: breakfast. Lunch: Well, if you go to a restaurant, you can find many tasty and healthy items. Dinner: Couldn't that be at home most evenings? If not, there are many good alternatives. Many restaurants offer some very good meals, and even at some fast-food places one can order meals that are modestly acceptable. Ethnic cuisine can be a great source of healthful tasty meals: Thai, Vietnamese, some Mexican (watch out for lard and vegetable shortening), Indian, and some Chinese (watch out for the deep-fried food and the sauces).

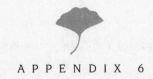

APPENDIX 6

Selected Bibliography

In the five-year preparation for this book, I consulted hundreds of articles, journals, and books. The major book sources are listed below.

Agatston, Arthur. *The South Beach Diet.* New York: Random House, 2003. A classic.

Balch, Phyllis, and James Balch. Prescription for Nutritional Healing. New York: Avery, 2000. An excellent encyclopedia of nutritional and dietary supplements, highly recommended for the home library.

Bensky, Dan, and Randall Barolet. *Chinese Herbal Medicine: Formulas and Strategies.* Seattle: Eastland Press, 1990.

Challem, Jack. *The Inflammation Syndrome*. Hoboken, N.J.: John Wiley and Sons, Inc., 2003. Challem is a science writer who has written a groundbreaking book about the importance of reducing internal inflammation to prevent chronic diseases like diabetes, arthritis, heart disease, and cancer. While Challem is a highly experienced writer, he is not a medical doctor or researcher. This has given him a perspective that insiders sometimes can't or don't want to have. While one might disagree with some of his opinions and points of view, this book puts the inflammation syndrome in clear perspective. I am indebted to Dr. Richard Roundtree of Boulder, Colorado, who mentioned this book in one of his lectures on detoxification.

Cloutier, Marissa, and Eve Adamson. *The Mediterranean Diet*. New York: Avon Books, 2004. This book is an excellent overview of one of the best nutritional programs on this planet, the basic diet of the Mediterranean people for hundreds of years. If all Americans ate like this, the pharmaceutical industry giants would have to shrink their waists.

Erasmus, Udo. *Fats That Heal, Fats That Kill*. Vancouver, Canada: Alive Books, 1993. A must-read for anyone who is interested in omega-3 fatty acids and health. This book should be required reading for all medical doctors.

Khalsa, Dharma Singh. *Food as Medicine: How to Use Diet, Vitamins, Juices, and Herbs for a Healthier, Happier, and Longer Life*. New York: Atria Books, 2003.

Lipman, Frank. *Total Renewal*. New York: Jeremy P. Tarcher, 2003. This book offers an intelligent and inspired synthesis of complementary, nutritional, and Western medicines.

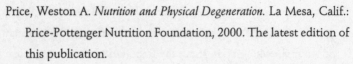

Price, Weston A. *Nutrition and Physical Degeneration.* La Mesa, Calif.: Price-Pottenger Nutrition Foundation, 2000. The latest edition of this publication.

Slaga, Thomas. *The Detox Revolution.* New York: McGraw-Hill, 2003. A prominent research scientist, Dr. Slaga put together an excellent overview of the modern view of detoxification, using foods and herbal medicines. His thoughts and ideas could revolutionize Western medicine, if it would focus on prevention and health promotion.

Stoll, Andrew L. *The Omega-3 Connection.* New York: Simon and Schuster, 2001. This book is an excellent overview of the value of omega-3 fatty acids in health. If you have any doubts about the validity of these healthful substances, read this book. They can positively alter moods, they can nourish the nervous system and brain, and they can reduce inflammation anywhere in the body.

Thondup, Tulku. *The Healing Power of the Mind.* Boston: Shambala, 1998. A practical and fascinating book about the techniques and philosophy of Tibetan medicine.

Walford, Roy L. *Maximum Lifespan.* New York: W. W. Norton, 1985.

Wilcox, Bradley J., D. Craig Wilcox, and Makoto Suzuki. *The Okinawa Diet Plan.* New York: Clarkson Potter, 2004. This is another superb nutrition book. Okinawa has more healthy elderly people than any other place on this planet. This book examines the diet and nutrition of these exceptionally healthy people.

Willet, Walter C. *Eat, Drink, and Be Healthy.* New York: Free Press, 2001. A sensible overview of healthy diet and nutrition that is a tonic after all the fad and specialty diet books. Other useful and sensible books about nutrition and health promotion include those by Dr. Andrew Weil and Dr. Dean Ornish.

Zimmermann, Michael. *Burgerstein's Handbook of Nutrition*. Zurich: Thieme Medical Publishers, 2001. A sound book on the role of nutrition in health care, written by an esteemed Swiss doctor.

For readers interested in a deep understanding of Oriental medicine, here is a good beginning:

Beinfield, Harriet, and Efrem Korngold. *Between Heaven and Earth: A Guide to Chinese Medicine*. New York: Ballantine Books, 1991.

Kaptchuk, Ted. *The Web That Has No Weaver*. New York: Congdon and Weed, 1983.

Pitchford, Paul. *Healing with Whole Foods*. Berkeley, Calif.: North Atlantic Books, 1993.

About the Author

Louis Vanrenen has operated his own clinic for
twenty-two years, focusing on acupuncture and
nutrition. He has studied with many pioneers of
acupuncture and holistic medicine, and his research
has taken him to Europe and Asia. Vanrenen teaches
extensively about disease prevention through health
promotion. Working full-time with patients, he helps
people optimize their health by supporting the health
of the whole body—with diet, exercise, acupuncture, and positive lifestyle changes. Currently he is
studying various approaches to cancer therapy and
working on a book about aging well. The father of
two adult children, Ariana and Gabriel, Vanrenen
lives in Massachusetts.